Thoughts on the Run
Glimpses of Wholistic Spirituality

Thomas E. Legere

Foreword

by

George Maloney, S.J.

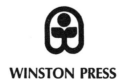

WINSTON PRESS

Cover design: Tom Egerman

Cover photograph: Robert Settles

Scripture texts used in this work are taken from the *New American Bible,* copyright © 1970 by the Confraternity of Christian Doctrine, Washington, D.C. Used by permission of the copyright owner. All rights reserved.

Library of Congress Catalog Card Number: 82-51162

ISBN: 0-86683-698-5

Printed in the United States of America.

5   4   3   2   1

Winston Press, Inc.
430 Oak Grove
Minneapolis, Minnesota 55403

To my family, who helped to teach me the beauty of life

Contents

Foreword . . . vii
Preface . . . ix

FAITH

True and False Disbelief . . . 1; As If . . . 2; Blues and Blahs
. . . 4; Am I My Brother's or Sister's Keeper? . . . 6; A
Young Man's Story . . . 7

INTERIORITY

A Swing Back to Noninvolvement . . . 11; A While Apart
. . . 13; Blessing in Disguise . . . 15; Our National Plague
. . . 16; Be Still . . . 18; Meditation: Christian or
Transcendental? . . . 20

PRAYER

The Jesus Prayer . . . 23; From Action to Prayer to Action
. . . 24; Does Prayer Work? . . . 26; Are Prayers
Answered? . . . 28

TURNINGS

The New Asceticism . . . 31; Who Is Saving Whom?
. . . 32; The Gift of Tears . . . 34; Religious Feelings
. . . 36; The Broken of Our World . . . 37; Repression Is
Regression . . . 39

GROPINGS

Mystery of Life . . . 43; What Are You Accomplishing?
. . . 44; Spiritual Work . . . 46; Joy Amid Suffering . . . 48;
Honesty Before God . . . 49; Today Is All There Is . . . 51;
Peaks, Plateaus, and Nadirs . . . 53; Dark Night . . . 55

LOVE

Self-Love Is Not Selfish . . . 57; Perfectionism . . . 58; That
Special Someone . . . 60; Pleasers . . . 62; Working with
Love . . . 64

CATHOLICISM

Why the Emptiness? . . . 67; Jesus' First Sermon . . . 68; Christian Americans . . . 69; Nice and . . . Unchallenging . . . 71; Used to Be . . . 72; Can You Say "Praise the Lord"? . . . 74; Words Are Like Fingers . . . 76

EXAMPLES

The Spunky Ones . . . 79; Well-Adjusted . . . 81; Sacristan Saint . . . 83; Prophetic Troublemakers . . . 84; Modern Heroes . . . 86

DEATH

"Mighty Matt" . . . 89; Not the Final Reality . . . 90; Vanity of Vanities . . . 92; A Beautiful Death . . . 94

BODY/MIND/SPIRIT

The Body . . . 97; Wholistic Medicine . . . 98; Fasting and Wholeness . . . 100; Listening to the Body . . . 102; Beyond Body Language . . . 104; Healing of Body and Spirit . . . 106

SELF-INTEGRATION

Science and Religion Together . . . 109; Jung at Heart . . . 110; God and Ego . . . 112; God and Superego . . . 114; Multiple Selves . . . 115

PROBLEMS

Seeking Religious Experience . . . 119; Stealing Fire . . . 120; False Psychics . . . 122; Negativism . . . 124; The Shadow Knows . . . 126; The Devil in Us . . . 127; Burnout . . . 129

PRACTICES

Spiritual Journal . . . 133; What Good Are Dreams? . . . 134; What's in a Dream? . . . 136; Run for Your Life . . . 138; Children of Light . . . 140; Positive Thinking . . . 141; Reclaiming Our Lives . . . 143

Foreword

Simple things in life are often the most difficult to talk about. How can you adequately describe the "ordinary" experience of a married man and woman who have lived with each other for fifty years? Or the pleasure of walking alone in a quiet woods as you "talk" with God? Or the simple joy of intimate conversation with a friend on a cold evening as you share a glass of wine before a warming fire?

God wishes us to meet him in all "ordinary" events of our lives. I guess that is why he puts us into so many routine and even banal situations, so that we can find him easily, around us and very near to us at all times.

This book is about finding God, by faith, in the ordinary things of life. It is about the simple relationship of our body, soul, and spirit. It is meant by the author, Father Thomas E. Legere, a diocesan priest of Camden, New Jersey, to be sparks of insight that will lead us to a greater share in the life that Jesus entered our broken world to bring us (John 10:10).

It is a privilege for me to introduce this work. I met the author at Fordham University when he was pursuing his master's degree in the Institute of Spirituality. The content and style seem so alarmingly simple and ordinary. I think this is the book's strong point. I plead with the reader to let these simple meditations create a movement in his or her heart, a yearning to become *whole* and fully *alive*.

Today much is being written about *wholistic* spirituality. It is an attempt to return to a more biblical view of us human beings, in accordance with the revelation of God's plan to share his own divine life with us. Too long we have sought to live our Christian lives according to an anthropology that comes more from Plato than from Jesus Christ.

Through dualism from such Hellenic rather than Semitic views, we have lived in a dichotomized world that has separated God from us, pitted spirit against matter, lined up the immortal soul opposite the mortal and sinful body. These essays are intended to give us a spiritual view that shows us not as made up of three parts—body, soul, and spirit—but as *whole* persons. We are in the process of becoming more healthy and full of God's life as we integrate our body, mind, and spirit and nurture our relationships with the material world around us, with other human beings, and ultimately with God.

The author draws from his years of study, vast reading, and, above all, his priestly ministry, to introduce the reader to a large range of topics from the Jesus prayer to dreams to false psychics. Yet underlying all of this rich and provocative material are the deep spiritual insights and personal faith of the author, which he so admirably and simply shares with his readers.

This is a disarmingly simple way of giving to you the reader a richness of spiritual direction. My prayer is added to the author's, that all who read this book may truly receive an increase in a richer faith, health, and life.

—George A. Maloney, S.J.

Preface

In 1972 I began writing a column for the *Catholic Star Herald*, the weekly newspaper of the Camden, New Jersey, diocese. Little did I realize at the time that the column would turn out to be a chronicle of a spiritual journey.

In the early columns most of my attention was centered on matters of social justice and institutional church reform. Gradually God began calling me to embark upon the inner journey, the very last thing I ever thought life would demand of me. Over the years, the change in my focus became apparent to the readers of the newspaper. Many persons remarked that they were fascinated to follow the saga of someone's journey within. This book is, for the most part, a selection of some of those columns that traced my journey to "the still point of the turning world" (T. S. Eliot).

Obviously no spirituality worth its salt can ever imply a narcissistic turning away from the real world. Indeed, I am more committed to social justice in church and society today than ever before. It is just that now, by God's grace, I have been able to discover a spiritual underpinning to social justice. This series of meditations will attempt to share some of the pains and insights and confusion and breakthroughs that have come to me in my struggle for firsthand experiential knowledge of the sacred.

A few turning points, in particular, stand out in my spiritual odyssey. In the summer of 1976, I went through a full blown existential crisis. My spiritual vision grew dim. My nerves were shot. And I developed a very painful psychosomatic illness: lower back pain.

Needless to say, I felt that my whole world was coming apart at the seams. I felt unable to cope and had no idea how or even if my crisis would ever be resolved. In a state of brokenness, when my ego had been all but shattered, I called out to the Higher Power from the very depths of my being. Until then, I had "said" prayers. But then I began to see that my life and sanity depended on surrendering to a dimension that was experientially unknown to me up until then. This was my "rebirth" experience and the beginning of an entirely new orientation of my life. My back pain was healed, my priorities got reorganized, and I discovered an inner peace that was, until then, only a theory to me.

During that same summer I also began studying for an M.A. in Spirituality at Fordham University. My experience at Fordham turned out to be one of life's greatest blessings for me. Under the tutelage of people like Prof. Ewert Cousins and Frs. George Maloney and Bernard Häring, I began to get in touch with the great spiritual wisdom of Christianity and other world religions. At Fordham I gained an understanding of the relationship between psychology and spirituality, and I gained the background necessary to begin a full-time ministry in spirituality.

As far as this work is concerned, I owe a debt of gratitude to Msgr. Salvatore Adamo, the former editor of the *Catholic Star Herald*. It was he who first encouraged me to write. Additional encouragement came from my family and friends. Without them I would never have had the courage to share my spiritual journey in the public forum. Thanks to Rosanne Bowen, Bonnie Piccioni, Mary Ann Scharlè, and Paula Wilson, who helped with the typing. Thanks, too, to William E. Jerman and Hermann Weinlick for their invaluable help in preparing the original manuscript for publication in book form.

FAITH

True and False Disbelief

"Well, if you get right down to it, the real reason I don't go to church is that I don't believe any of it. I don't believe that Christ was the Son of God, and I don't think the church has anything to do with the way I live my life. Period."

At long last, I had finally come upon someone who was rejecting the gospel for a logical reason—namely, he did not believe a word of it. He did not believe that Christ was anyone special, and he did not believe that the Christian way of life was what he was looking for.

This person did not blame his lack of faith on the fact that Father McGillicuddy had hollered at him in confession back in the third grade; he did not blame it on the fact that someone had cut him off on the way out of the church parking lot, or the fact that he might happen to prefer Latin to English, or the allegation that the Vatican is wealthy, or the fact that a priest he used to know had gotten married.

The excuses we come up with for evading the central challenge of the gospel are innumerable. We love to find one peripheral issue after another in order to avoid facing the really big questions: Does life have any meaning? Was Jesus someone special? Is the teaching of Jesus worth following?

It is understandable, I suppose, that some persons feel alienated from the church because of an isolated incident in their past. No one is left with a favorable impression after being berated in the confessional or being insulted at a Holy Name meeting. We must realize, however, that rejecting Christ because of a shortcoming of one of the church's ministers or members is a first-class cop-out.

When we have to face the Lord at the end of our lives, it will do us no good whatever to blame our lack of faith on the pastor

or the president of the Holy Name Society. God will ask us
what we thought about his Son and whether or not we lived
according to the gospel. Pointing an accusatory finger at others
as a rationalization for our own poor behavior will be an
exercise in futility.

One of the flimsiest excuses for rejecting Christianity was
offered to me by a man recently. He said he is a nonbeliever
because he prayed for a big increase in salary and he never
received it. Another man said he was rejecting the church
because he once saw a priest wearing a sweatshirt. As bizarre
and far-out as these examples are, they are not products of my
imagination.

When I dialogue with others about Jesus and his message,
sometimes I run into genuine unbelievers. I can at least respect
them, even if I do not agree with their conclusions. These rare
individuals feel that loving our neighbor, especially our
enemy, is nothing but hopeless idealism. Or they believe that
there is no need to look beyond the limits of science for a
solution to the problems that plague humankind. Or they
believe that Jesus of Nazareth was a very holy man, but not the
Son of God. For these reasons they choose to reject
Christianity.

There is no way I can agree with the conclusions of these
honest-to-goodness unbelievers, but at least we can carry on a
fruitful exchange of ideas. We are speaking the same language, and I admire them because they are facing up to the real
questions in life.

I feel nothing but pity, however, for the cop-out artists who
blame their disbelief on everything except their own lack of
faith in Jesus.

As If

We will never experience God unless we first of all act "as if"
God exists.

For a skeptical society, that is a bitter pill to swallow. We
refuse to believe anything unless it can be scientifically dem-

onstrated to us. We will believe in a personal God only when the evidence is totally convincing.

Belief in God is not illogical. It makes a lot of sense. But the evidence is persuasive rather than convincing.

To be able to experience God fully, we must learn to let go of our worship of reason and logic. Some of the best things in life are beyond reason and logic. How can we explain love? What makes a painting by Chagall or Van Gogh so powerful? How does one speak logically about laughter or a pretty girl or a striking sunset?

In order to experience God, we must let our hearts lead our heads. This is a rough assignment for us who value "head knowledge" so highly. But all the great religions of the world are in complete agreement on this point. Reason and logic, however important they may be, are not enough for us to experience the God within.

The process by which we let go of a fixation on reason and logic and step into the unknown is what we call faith. Faith is neither blind nor irrational. It questions and evaluates, but always after the fact. In other words, by faith you trust enough to give it a try and act "as if" God is alive. The proof of the pudding is in the tasting. If it does not help us, we drop it. But unless we give it a shot, we will never find out whether or not it helps us.

Faith is something like the attitude we need in order to enjoy the theater. If we approach a performance solely from our head, we will never really appreciate it. We will spend our time telling ourselves that the scenery is fake, the stage is not really in a foreign country, and Peter Pan is not really flying across the stage. To say the least, we will totally miss the point of what is going on. In order to fully appreciate the performance, we will have to suspend momentarily our critical faculties and act "as if" it is all really happening.

Admittedly this is risky business. At least with our reason and our logic we know where we are, and we feel sure of ourselves. This faith business seems to be asking us to let go of that security blanket and plunge into the darkness.

Almost invariably, those who have had the courage to take the plunge feel that it was the best move they ever made. *And they discover the divine paradox that darkness really is light.*

We will never discover any of this until we let go and dare to act "as if" it is all true.

Blues and Blahs

Depression is the nation's number one emotional illness. In a recent year, 125,000 Americans were hospitalized with it, another 200,000 were treated by professionals, and God only knows how many others had it but sought no professional help.

Everyone experiences depression at times. Of course, it may only be a mild case of the "blahs." But often it progresses to the "weeps" and sometimes even to despondency or despair.

Depression is no respecter of persons. Everyone from blue-collar workers to homemakers to doctors to clergy may at times experience it.

To feel depressed is no sin. According to Fr. Benedict Groeschel, director of spiritual development for the archdiocese of New York, even Jesus manifested the symptoms of depression when he wept openly over the city of Jerusalem.

Apparently the causes of depression are legion. They include anger, guilt, fear, fatigue, physical illness, pain, malnutrition, aging, misuse of medication, diabetes, hormonal imbalance, anemia, disappointment, and lack of self-esteem.

The big question is how to treat this debilitating illness. If you go to the doctor, he or she may treat you with drug therapy. Such therapy has done wonders—but it treats the *symptom* rather than the *cause*. In some extreme cases physicians recommend electrotherapy, a controversial form of treatment with obvious, scary drawbacks. The average garden-variety depressive can usually be greatly helped by psychotherapy. Going to a professional to help pinpoint the cause is necessary in some cases. But often just talking over problems with a pastor or good friend is sufficient for the time being.

But there is a form of spiritual therapy available to all Christians that is much more effective, in certain cases, than drug therapy, electrotherapy, or psychotherapy. I am referring to the power of Jesus Christ.

There is a whole theology available to explain theoretically this power of Jesus. But people are never impressed by theory. Only experience seems to be able to move hearts. And it is the experience of countless millions of Christians over the last two thousand years that Christ is able to cure physical, spiritual, and emotional difficulties, including depression.

It would be fruitless to argue the previous paragraph on a theoretical basis. Come to think of it, one person's experience will not necessarily convince someone else. The power of Christ is just one of those self-validating kinds of things that happen in life sometimes.

Until a few years ago, I had never experienced depression. When it came, I felt as if the bottom had fallen out of my life. At a loss as to what to do, I began to think about Christ with praise and thanksgiving. Gradually I could feel my blue funk lifting. Finally it disappeared.

The depression returned once more later, but it disappeared again when I determined to get out of myself and praise God for the sun and the stars and even the clouds. Such an experience does not prove anything, of course, but it was good enough for me at the time.

The key to this process of spiritual therapy is faith. Not faith in a collection of rules and regulations and doctrines, but faith in the power of Jesus. If we do not believe in his spiritual power, we will never call on him. So what do we do now? Crease our brows, clench our fists, and try to summon up some faith? No, that does not work.

The next time you feel down and out, just try to be aware that there may be a solution you have never tried before. It has to do with trusting a power greater than your own to lift you out of your depression back to reality.

Am I My Brother's or Sister's Keeper?

The Italians are the most tolerant human beings I have ever met. That is probably why an uncharacteristic incident that I witnessed one summer in Italy upset me so much.

I was standing in a crowded, second-class train going from Naples to Rome. A few yards away from me there was a group of young soldiers, most of whom were probably not more than nineteen years of age. They seemed like a nice enough group of young men, but they did something that upset me very much. They started making fun of an old man who was on the train with us. They made fun of his old clothes, his old suitcase, and his comical dialect.

Looking back on my own life, I must admit that ten or so years earlier I probably would have been right in there with those soldiers making fun of the old man. Young men sometimes show a certain propensity to cruelty. But as a grown man I was sickened by that spectacle. I elbowed my way over to the soldiers and persuaded them to leave the old man alone.

I have been thinking about that incident quite a bit lately. I have been asking myself what happened in my life to make me change my values so much over the years. And I have to conclude that I have changed because of my faith in Jesus Christ.

I really believe that Jesus is my brother and all human beings are my brothers and sisters. All persons are equal in the sight of God. All persons deserve my respect despite their age, or their education, or their nationality.

This may sound like coming out in favor of apple pie and motherhood. But if you think about it awhile, it is really dynamite. Everyone in the world is my brother or sister. This belief enables me to transcend ethnic backgrounds, economic situations, political ideologies. It is truly an insight that liberates.

Most persons seem to do relatively well in treating their families, friends, and neighbors with respect. Where they commonly falter is when someone starts talking about persons of different racial backgrounds. That is "knot in the stomach" time for most of us. And when you try to go one step further and ask someone to love *everybody*—from illegal immigrants to unwed mothers—they begin to develop a gastrointestinal ulcer or want to start swinging at you.

The seeming innocuous statement, "Everyone is my brother or sister," is then seen to be not so harmless after all. In fact, if an individual believes this statement and tries to live according to it, chances are he or she will be labeled everything from a naive dreamer to a communist.

We might get upset when we see someone pushing around one of our neighbors or when we hear young persons making fun of the elderly. But, for some strange reason, it does not seem to bother us much at all when we read of thousands starving to death in India, or being killed in Central America or Southeast Asia.

The poets and prophets of the church point out to us our inconsistencies. They keep reminding us that if we are followers of Jesus, then we must indeed be our brother's and sister's keeper. Too many of us wish they would go away and leave us in peace.

There are many "negotiable" aspects of our faith, but one of the absolutely nonnegotiable tenets is that everyone who lives on planet Earth is our brother or sister.

What we think of that unqualified statement, and how well we live it, will be touchstones of our worth as followers of Jesus.

A Young Man's Story

This is the story of a friend of mine who became a Christian. He is typical of those intelligent young persons born in the 1940s and 1950s who have had to struggle for faith in a world that has ceased to believe in the reality of the spiritual.

Let me call my friend Ted. His mother was a Catholic and his father an agnostic. His father was very intelligent and had a way of making Christianity seem totally ridiculous. Ted had a good relationship with his mother but felt that her religious ideas were somewhat naive.

Ted was a brilliant student, but when his father went bankrupt in business, Ted was forced to drop out of school to help support the family. He bummed around for a year and went the whole promiscuity route.

Luckily, a wealthy neighbor who recognized his talent lent him enough money to resume his schooling. Ted went back to school and moved in with his lover. She bore him a son. All the while he remained at the top of his class. When he graduated from college he was given a teaching fellowship at a local university.

Ted's "inner journey" was as chaotic as the outward events in his life. He tried practically everything, including astrology and Eastern religion, but he was skeptical of the claims of Christianity. He examined them briefly, but was turned off by the simplistic approach of Christianity, especially the Scriptures. He just could not handle all that stuff about Adam and Eve and the apple and the like.

The first time Ted ever considered the possibility that Christianity was even remotely believable was when he met an intelligent priest who was able to speak his language. This priest explained to him a few things about the proper interpretation of the Scriptures. He also gave him a solid philosophical basis for understanding the principal teachings of Christianity.

It was at this point that God broke dramatically into Ted's life. He had a very powerful "religious experience" that for the first time gave him primary knowledge of the realm of the spiritual. According to sociologist Andrew Greeley, many Americans privately admit to having had similar religious experiences. It is just that they usually dismiss them because they are afraid that others, especially their clergy, will think they are crazy if they talk about their experiences.

Ted was not able to dismiss his religious experience; it was too real to him. He also was not able to dismiss the explanations of Christianity that the priest had given him. But he was too independent to submit to anyone else. He enjoyed free sex and free thinking too much. He was very much afraid that becoming a Christian would end all that.

The pressure of trying to reconcile what he now knew in his heart to be right with what he did not want to give up finally became too much for him. After developing a psychosomatic illness, he had a nervous breakdown.

According to Thomas Merton, a conversion experience can correspond to what doctors call a nervous breakdown. In any event Ted hit rock bottom and felt he had nowhere else to turn. As a last resort, he called out in his heart to Jesus Christ.

That decision was the beginning of a whole new direction in his life. At first he still had some doubts, but the healing experience of Jesus in his mind and heart was so real to him that he could not deny it. Ted eventually straightened out his life and then shocked everyone by entering the seminary and being ordained a priest.

Should I tell you Ted's real name? Why not? He is St. Augustine, born in the year 354, a man who went on to become a bishop, a theologian, and a great teacher of the church.

Is there anyone who is beyond conversion? Beyond recovery?

INTERIORITY

A Swing Back to Noninvolvement

Recently the undergraduates of Ursinus College near Philadelphia got their name in the *Guinness Book of Records* by assembling the world's largest hot dog. This is the kind of thing happening on college campuses these days. Just think, back in the 1960s we had students marching for civil rights, protesting the war in Indochina, and demanding a say in the political process.

Most Americans are probably overjoyed that so many of our students and the populace at large have quit doing much about the ills of society. Personally, the nation's change in priorities gives me a sick feeling in the pit of my stomach. But I guess the swing back to noninvolvement was inevitable. Why? Whatever happened to the Great Society and the nation's finest aspirations? What blighted the "greening of America"?

It seems to me our tragic flaw was that most of us were on an "ego trip" inasmuch as we tried to do things ourselves. There was not enough trust in God involved; it was all "us" and our self-righteous calls for reform. There was little depth to the social activism. It did not come from the wellsprings of the human spirit.

Consequently, after a few short years, most activists grew tired. They did not see instant results, so they became frustrated, detached, and disillusioned. Their little projects did not work out the way they had hoped. So they turned back to preoccupation with self.

Some time ago, I saw Joan Baez interviewed on one of the TV talk shows. The interviewer asked why we do not hear much from her these days. He wanted to know why her voice, which once rang out clearly for social reform, is now so silent.

Ms. Baez replied that she was taking a six-month sabbatical

from social involvement. She was trying to pace herself because she saw what had happened to her friends. She said, "Just about everyone has given up. I don't want the same thing to happen to me, too."

Most have grown weary of social involvement and are now preoccupied with old *numero uno.* It seems that everybody is "getting their head together" these days. This takes the form of Silva Mind Control, Arica, EST, transcendental meditation, biorhythms, and God knows what all else. You name it; all your personal needs can be met by the supermarket approach to human personality development.

This preoccupation with self has prompted one psychologist to name our age "The New Narcissism": endless navel-gazing with a consequent blocking out of the real problems of human concern.

Does the renewed interest in Christian prayer and inner development fit this description? Not really, at least not with genuine Christian prayer. The renewal of interest in prayer may indeed be prompted by the same nervous exhaustion that characterized the end of the 1960s. But there is one crucial difference. Authentic Christian prayer will not allow us to remain on the level of self.

When we have an authentic encounter with the Trinity, we meet a living God who sends us back to wash the feet of our brothers and sisters. The Christian life is as much concerned with our neighbor as it is with God. We respond to God's radical love for us with a radical concern for the needs of others.

Any religious movement that shuns the problems of the real world should be suspect. If your prayer is just an escape that makes you feel good, it most emphatically is not authentic Christian prayer.

The 1970s were a mixed bag. Some of our contemporaries lived their lives on the surface. For them I had little respect. Some went deep into themselves and remained shut up there. These persons were on the road to disillusionment.

But some of us have been driven to our knees in a search for

the living God. If we find him, both we and the world will be
better off as a result.

A While Apart

Even accompanied by twenty-nine superactive teenagers, I
still found it a very peaceful weekend. It was peaceful because
all of us were able to get some perspective on our daily
problems.

Our youth group's "weekend in Christian living" came just
in the nick of time for me. The tragic murder of a fellow priest,
as well as my witnessing the near-fatal heart attack of one of
our parishioners, had my nerves on edge. The kids had their
own set of problems. They were happy to get away, too.

As the cars pulled into our refuge in the Pocono Mountains
(an old farmhouse belonging to one of the parishioners), we all
felt a great burden lifting from our shoulders.

On this plot of ground we were free to be ourselves; we
were temporarily liberated from society's pressures. No one
worried about how we dressed, whether our hair was
combed, or whether it is socially acceptable to lie down on a
hillside and stare at the stars. We would have time enough to
worry about social conventions all year long. This was a
weekend to celebrate the fact that we are all children of God,
brothers and sisters to one another.

This was the fifth year that I had taken the teenagers to the
rolling hills of Pennsylvania. Never had things clicked as well
as they did that year. The kids were hungry to discover how
they fit into the plan of God's creation. They spent time by
themselves, dialoguing with others, praying, playing, sleep-
ing, eating, helping one another, coming to know better the
Lord and one another.

How it happened I am not exactly sure, but by Sunday
afternoon the twenty-nine teenagers and seven adults had
come together in a real community of love. We now appreciated one another on an entirely different level from what had

been before. The hackneyed word "community" was no longer an empty concept for us. We knew what it meant by
firsthand experience.

None of the discoveries of that weekend would have taken
place without the perspective gained by stepping back from
the rat race for a while.

This, of course, has been the church's rationale over the
centuries in encouraging persons to make retreats. Stepping
back for a while is a sound principle in spirituality, going back
to the days of the fathers of the church who went off by
themselves to the Egyptian desert along the Nile. Jesus himself
made time in his busy schedule to take frequent trips to the
desert to make sure his motives and actions were in accord
with the will of his Father.

Even though we know an occasional retreat makes good
sense, somehow with an upbringing influenced by the American work ethic, we often feel guilty about taking the time off.
Laypersons and sometimes even priests succeed in convincing
themselves that they are too busy to spend the necessary time
on their own interior, spiritual lives. In reality, no one is too
busy to spend some time with God.

Singles and married persons without children generally
have an easier time getting away for a weekend than do
parents. They can go to a retreat house or make a Cursillo and
not have to worry about the kids. But this spiritual perspective
is so important for one's growth as a Christian that fathers and
mothers too should do everything within their power to try to
arrange it so that they can make a retreat every so often, either
together or separately.

If, as sometimes happens, this is absolutely impossible, then
we can at least arrange for daily mini-retreats: ten-minute
pockets of time when we can be alone and give the Lord a
chance to get through to us.

Some may have the impression that it is easy for me to say
this inasmuch as I am a parish priest. However, I think my
schedule would compare with anyone else's. We are all busy.
But with so much at stake, busyness is no excuse. If Jesus

managed to make time, so can we.

Blessing in Disguise

It would seem that one of the worst things ever to happen to this country was the whole drug scene. But guess what? God has made something good come out of even that mess.

First of all, it has introduced millions of secularized Americans to the experience of altered states of consciousness. Once a person has been on an LSD trip or even just mellowed out on marijuana, there is no way that you will ever be able to convince him or her that there is only one way to experience reality.

Many young persons today are returning to prayer and meditation principally because they now know for a fact that there is more to life than meets the eye. Their dabbling with drugs has turned out to be a blessing in disguise. God has a way of doing things like that. He takes even our mistakes and fits them into his eternal plan.

Of course, an altered state of consciousness is not in itself prayer. A person can be experiencing all sorts of feelings without coming closer to God. But at least it is a start. Millions of Americans now at least believe there is such a thing as spiritual reality. They can compare some of the things that have happened to them while on drug trips to some of the sensations and feelings of our mystics, who were able by prayer to get down below the surface of life.

Meditation takes a person down through the same levels of consciousness that drugs do, but there are all sorts of differences, too. For one thing, meditation is safe. One can come back to the surface at will. There is little danger that a person will get lost in the subconscious.

The safety factor goes by the name of Jesus Christ. With him as our companion on the inner way, we have nothing whatever to fear. There is no force in the subconscious that can overwhelm the Son of God. He is strong. He gives us a reference point. We do not make the journey alone.

With drugs you are all by yourself. If you get lost down there, you could quite literally lose your mind. You can get so far along the inner way that you forget how to get back to home base.

Many artists and poets have tried to penetrate beneath the surface of life without Christ and some of them have had, to say the least, a really bad trip. To cite only a few examples, Hart Crane jumped off a ship, Ernest Hemingway blew his brains out, and Edgar Allan Poe drank himself to death.

Other artists and poets, such as Dante and T. S. Eliot, made the inner journey in the company of the living God. As a result they were personally enriched and they made a more lasting contribution to humankind's understanding of itself than did those artists who were swallowed up by their subconscious.

To many moderns, all this is a lot of mumbo jumbo. They think artists and poets are weird anyway, and they have even less time for authentic religion. For such folks, drinking beer and watching the tube are what life is all about.

We should not put down such individuals. They are where they are, for the most part, through no fault of their own. But we should not imitate them either.

There is more to life than you can see on the surface. Spiritually sensitive persons have always known this. A whole generation has recently discovered it, in God's providence, by the use of mind-expanding drugs.

How we got to where we are is immaterial. But where we go from here is crucially important. Spiritual gourmets will continue to use their experiences for their own ego glorification. The truly religious man or woman will keep on moving in pursuit of the living God.

Our National Plague

One of the best things about being in Italy is eating. The meals there are real events in themselves, something to look forward to. The food is superdelicious, of course, but the *best* part is sitting down with one's friends for two or three hours and sharing one's thoughts and personality with those at table. If you go to a restaurant, the waiter does everything he can to help you relax and make the meal enjoyable. Nothing is rushed.

The Italians and some of the other Europeans may be behind us technologically, but they know how to live better. They may not have electric toothbrushes and microwave ovens, but who cares? They know how to emphasize what is more important in life.

I will never forget my reintroduction to the American scene after four years of living the sane, leisurely pace of the Italians. I had just arrived at Kennedy Airport in New York. I sat down at a lunch counter there, casually looking over the menu, when an impatient waitress barked, "Whaddya want, buddy, a hamburger?" I cringed.

One of the most important things in life is taking time to worship God. This can be done both privately and communally. Ideally, there should be room in a person's life for both the more private and the more public nurturing of one's spirit.

That is the ideal. In America, however, we are too busy for this prayer stuff. We have jobs to hold down, churches to build, grass to cut, cobwebs to remove, and Monday-night football to watch. We are very busy.

In the process, of course, we are starving our spirits. We give them no nourishment whatsoever. That is why so many Americans are tense, drink too much, pop too many pills, walk the malls to kill time, watch the "soaps," and never take time to smell the roses.

It would seem that the very minimum step in counteracting our spiritual lethargy would be to participate in one meaningful religious ritual each week. This would at least increase the possibility of some religious encounter on a more frequent basis.

We are, of course, too busy to do that. The number of the "unchurched" has risen dramatically. Millions have decided that they do not need religious ritual any more. If they were replacing this lack with some personal, private devotion, it might not be so bad. But, honestly, are they?

Those who still come to church are making an effort, but it seems that even many of them are being shortchanged. Instead of a relaxing, leisurely approach (essential for any religious experience to take place), clergy frequently rush through the ritual as if finishing on time were the number one priority.

According to recent popes, there should be fewer Sunday services so that worshipers can acquire a keener sense of community and community prayer. But in many parishes worshipers are rushed in and rushed out again, deprived of any chance for an unhurried, in-depth prayer experience. The major consideration seems to be how fast the parking lot can be cleared for the next Mass.

Yes, this assembly line is wrong and counterproductive. No wonder our spirits are not being nourished. The average American watches four hours of television per day, but we are too busy to spend fifteen minutes in prayer. And our one spiritual oasis, our one hour of prayer per week, becomes a thirty-five or forty minute religious exercise—out of deference to the parking lot.

We are reaping what we are sowing. Despite Pope Pius XII's decrying of the heresy of activism, it is our national plague. The bubonic plague killed only the body; our plague kills the spirit.

Be Still

Without significant moments of silence, progress in the spiritual life is a delusion.

Silence is very important in Zen Buddhism, Taoism and Islam. It used to be important in Christianity. That was because the early church was aware of how important silence was to Jesus. But somewhere along the way we got detoured into an overactive brand of religion, especially we in the United

States.

Catholic Church members fell victim to the American "can-do," "go-get-'em" lifestyle that so many in this country were living. Bricks and mortar were symbols of success. Pastors were valued for how many buildings they put up and how fast they paid off their debt. Sisters would make Wonder Woman wonder as they handled seventy, eighty, even ninety children in a class. The laity, too, organized themselves into all sorts of action-oriented clubs and sodalities.

Fortunately, the Catholic liturgy offered profound, meaningful moments of silence in which the average person could come into contact with the living God. But now even that is gone. As beautiful as the revised liturgy is, it is too wordy. It is all so logical and conscious that we have snuffed out that mystical, meditative milieu that used to mean so much to us.

Now we Catholics have joined the rest of society as we work ourselves into our graves to achieve, accomplish, acquire, and impress. With so much to do, we have no time for the "luxury" of silence. We are glutted with news and noise from the moment we are awakened by the clock-radio until the moment we hit the sack after watching the evening news.

The result of this lifestyle is that we do not even know who we are anymore. We bounce back and forth like ping-pong balls, reacting to situations rather than freely initiating what we do. In the process, everyone seems to be going through an identity crisis.

We need to change gears, put on the brakes, so that we can begin living instead of just existing. We need to learn how to live as human beings instead of as robots. None of this will ever be accomplished until we have learned to be comfortable with silence and solitude.

We instinctively fear silence and solitude because we know that when the din of the crowd fades into the background, we will finally have to face ourselves. The barriers that we have so carefully erected between our conscious and our sub-conscious will come crashing down like the walls of Jericho. When that happens, we come face-to-face with our own

sinfulness and duplicity. Such an experience can be overwhelming. We will do almost anything to avoid it.

Maybe that was the rationale behind the old adage "an idle
mind is the devil's workshop." To be sure, there is a lot of
devilment inside us. After all, we carry in our psyches the
cumulative baggage of our primitive ancestors. We are not all
that far removed from the Stone Age.

But if we can hang in there and courageously face the scary
part of who we are, sooner or later our fundamental beauty
will begin to shine forth, too. And we shall discover that our
inner beauty is not really us; it is Christ. And once that dawns
on us, we are saved. Saved from what? From our fears and
insecurities that cause defensive and obnoxious behavior.

Today thousands of Christians are rising above their herd
instincts, crossing their inner desert, and at least getting a
glimpse of the Promised Land. But none of that will ever
happen to a person until he or she first of all gets the courage to
be still.

Meditation: Christian or Transcendental?

According to a recent Gallup poll, there are over six million
Americans who practice transcendental meditation. Many of
these six million are Christians. These Christians have been
ripped off. There are techniques of meditation within our
tradition that are safer, more rewarding, and a lot cheaper than
the $125 initiation fee the Maharishi and his disciples charge.

The reason so many Americans are involved in TM is that
the side effects of the discipline are quite beneficial. After
spending a weekend learning the technique, devotees spend
twenty minutes each evening letting their minds "transcend"
the outer world and slip down into their subconscious.

This "instant retreat" from the stresses and strains of our
daily world enables many individuals to calm down, lower
their blood pressure, improve their memory or even their
ability to reason. Most followers of TM experience one or

more of these beneficial side effects.

So where is the danger in all of this? If individuals just do their twenty minutes and never go any deeper than that, there probably is not much danger. But whenever you are monkeying around with the mind, particularly the subconscious, you had better know what you are doing. The subconscious can be treacherous territory in which to travel. It is easy to lose your bearings.

In the subconscious you see previously hidden ramifications of life. Sometimes this can be scary. Many poets and artists who were able to get beneath the surface of life (into the subconscious) could not handle what they found once they got there.

The main reason so many of our poets and artists are overcome by the subconscious is that often they are not following a spiritual path. They are dabbling with the mind and exploring the subconscious. As Morton Kelsey is always saying, the spiritual journey is not for dabblers. It is serious business.

This is the major danger I see with TM. It is not taught with any spiritual basis to it. Indeed, its proponents go out of their way to dissociate TM from any religious path. As a consequence, it is open to anyone. For most people there probably will not be any difficulty with it. But if someone gets involved who has either emotional problems or the wrong motivation, other problems could develop.

With Christian meditation, we are in a completely different realm. Here one does not even enter into meditation without trust in the power of the Risen Christ. One is not going into emptiness, but into the Presence. One is not exploring the subconscious out of curiosity. One is in search of the Living God.

Of course, even here it is essential that the Christian be of sound mental and emotional health before getting too deeply into meditation. It is also often advisable to get some guidance beforehand from someone experienced in meditative techniques.

But once the appropriate precautions have been taken, then full speed ahead. And why not? Christians believe that at the depth of everything, including their own minds, lies the Trinity. They are not afraid to travel through the subconscious, because they know where they are going. They are not just going into the void or the abyss. They are in God's temple and they know that meditation is leading them to an encounter with the Living God.

So if you have $125 to burn and are so confident of yourself that you are convinced you could never lose your bearings in life, then go take a course in TM. But if you want to explore the depths of your mind with Jesus (instead of the Maharishi) as your guru, then seek out a priest, a sister, or a layperson who knows something about Christian meditation. You will end up with the same benefits as those who practice TM, but, besides just "getting your head together," you will also be getting your soul together.

PRAYER

The Jesus Prayer

To some the Jesus prayer seems like only a fad in Christian prayer, but not to those who understand its rationale and inner dynamics. The simple recitation of the formula "Lord Jesus, Son of God, have mercy on me, a sinner" has touched an exposed nerve in Western spirituality, which this prayer is uniquely capable of affecting.

The power of this prayer comes from its reliance on the name of Jesus. Members of the early church were quite conscious of the uniqueness of that name: "It is the Name of this same Jesus; it is faith in that Name which has cured this man" (Acts 3:16).

The repetition of a religious formula over and over again in order to focus one's concentration is nothing new. The Eastern religions have employed mantras for centuries. Nor is there anything new in seeking inner peace by merging the empirical ego with the All.

What sharply distinguishes the Jesus prayer from other spiritual exercises that employ the recitation of mantras is belief in the power of the name of Jesus. The repetition of the name Jesus is much more than an aid in concentration. It is a powerful means of healing the total person.

The Jesus prayer can be traced back to a fourth century Syrian monk whom historians have named Pseudo-Macarius. An orthodox renaissance of the prayer was developed by St. Gregory of Sinai in the fourteenth century.

Although it has been around for centuries, lately the Jesus prayer has burst forth into the prayer life of western Christians with surprising suddenness. Perhaps this is because the West has become so intellectual, rational, conceptual, and rigid in its prayer forms that it is very much in need of this valuable contribution from the East.

What is its secret? What is the reason for its popularity? Simply stated, the Jesus prayer is more than just a prayer. It is a way of life. It is a way of synchronizing body, mind, and spirit under the lordship of Jesus.

When this dynamic takes place, there frequently develops a sense of communal sinfulness. The person who prays gradually acquires a sense of compunction not just for his or her own sin, but for the sin of all men and women living and dead. The one who prays the Jesus prayer becomes, in a sense, a cosmic person. He or she takes on responsibility for the human race and intercedes on its behalf.

Besides the sense of union with the human family, another effect of the Jesus prayer is a sense of union with nature. Seeing the unity of all of creation leads one to a sense of reverence for God's creation.

But the most significant reason for the popularity of the Jesus prayer is that it gives persons an immediate experience of God's presence. They have heard for years that God dwells inside of them. Praying the Jesus prayer makes that teaching an experienced reality. And the wonder of the dynamic is that meeting Jesus is only the beginning of a full life with the Trinity. Jesus leads one to the loving Father and gives one a palpable experience of the Spirit.

Much more could, of course, be said. In fact many books have been written on the subject. We are dealing here with much more than a Christian mantra. We are dealing with the same reality Peter expressed in Acts when he came to the conclusion there is no other name by which we can be saved.

From Action to Prayer to Action

A few years ago Pope John Paul II met with leaders of the Catholic Church in Latin America. His remarks to these bishops marked him as a man of vision and profound spirituality. He spoke of the need for redistribution of wealth, land reform, and human rights. He could not have been more specific.

Yet the press jumped on Pope John Paul because he did not summon the church to join forces with Marxism to accomplish these worthy goals. In no way did the pope downplay the need for the church to be vitally concerned with the plight of the poor. However, he realized that a prayerful person, in touch with the white-hot fire of the Holy Spirit, is a far more effective instrument of long-term justice than is a doctrinaire Marxist.

Political ideologies come and go. They all have their flaws—especially Marxism, which denies the spiritual nature of human beings. Authentic Christianity is here to stay and will continue to be the most profound statement ever uttered about the interplay of the human and the divine.

The pope did not think Marxism was too radical; he thought it was not radical enough. Only God-filled persons will ever succeed in making this world the way it is supposed to be.

Some moderns are surprised when they hear of the interconnection between prayer and social action. They have always thought that prayer was synonymous with escapism. Actually, nothing could be further from the truth. Authentic prayer always leaves one with a sense of compassion for persons. Those who have no desire to serve and love the world have not had an authentic Christian prayer experience.

The world learned this lesson again from Thomas Merton. When he went the agnostic-to-Catholic-to-monastery route, he was held up as an example to young Catholics. The Bill Buckleys of the country positively drooled over such a fine example of Catholic spirituality. Merton had turned his back on the world to seek the things of God. How noble!

But then a funny thing happened to Tom Merton. His prayer naturally led him to be concerned again with political life. In fact, according to Merton, all prayer is political; it always has social ramifications.

At first, Merton began to speak out on civil rights. When he predicted in the 1950s that we would eventually have race riots in our cities, some thought he must have been eating too much Trappist cheese. When he took a stand on the Vietnam war, the Bill Buckleys publicly disowned him.

His most prophetic expression of global concern had to do with his interest in Buddhism. Merton was not even satisfied with reaching out to his compatriots in the political arena. He wanted to reach out to the world spiritually. When he left his monastery to visit the Dalai Lama, his superiors thought he should check out a psychiatrist on the way there.

Merton cared about the blacks and the Vietnamese and the Buddhists because he was a prayerful man. This is how he once described a person with a bogus, uncaring spirituality: "As long as he can be by himself and nurse that warm interior sweetness of rest in the center of himself—which may well be only an illusory shadow of true contemplation—the whole world can fall to pieces and the monastery with it, for all he cares."

Persons like Pope John Paul II and Thomas Merton are dangerous. When we foolishly criticize such giants, I just hope that the likes of John Paul and Thomas Merton are patient with us. They know that the Holy Spirit is not here to sprinkle holy water on the status quo.

Does Prayer Work?

A friend may ask us, "Say a prayer for me, will ya?" And we quickly respond, "Sure."

But do we believe the prayer will accomplish anything? Do we ever get around to saying the prayer? Does prayer work? Or is it just one of those pious leftovers from our Christian tradition?

A compromise answer would be that praying for one another is effective when the other person knows we are praying for him or her. The knowledge that another person loves and supports us can enable us to transcend obstacles and help us to persevere.

But this answer is a bit of a hedge. It is a way of taking prayer (which has been considered a powerful spiritual reality for millennia) and explaining it away as a form of positive reinforcement.

To get down to the basic question: if someone is praying for us but we do not know about it, does anything happen that could possibly change the course of our life? It has been the experience of Christians for the last two thousand years that praying for others is definitely effective. Note the all-important word "experience." Belief in the effectiveness of prayer was not dreamed up by a group of cardinals meeting in a smoke-filled room at the Vatican. It has been the universal experience of millions of Christians who have gone before us that something indeed happens when we pray for others.

Not everyone born before the year 1900 was a total idiot. If our Christian predecessors did not experience "answers" to their prayers, then, surely, they would have done something more productive with their time.

But some modern persons are incredibly arrogant. Because we have invented electric can-openers and uniformly-shaped potato chips, we somehow feel that we are superior to all those who have gone before us. Many twentieth-century know-it-alls casually dismiss spiritual giants such as Jesus, the Buddha, and Mohammed as sincere individuals who were operating out of a primitive worldview that persons no longer take seriously.

But wisdom always wins out in the end. In fact, some of our greatest skeptics are now beginning to take another look at the power of prayer. For many, their reexamination of the power of prayer began with plants. Yes, *plants*. Nonbelievers started noticing that their household plants grew better when they "talked" to them. Whatever you want to call it, some force was being directly transmitted from individuals to their plants.

Some scientists decided to examine this whole phenomenon under laboratory conditions. It was their unexpected (to say the least) finding that persons could indeed affect the health of plants, even across great distances, by positive or negative feelings they directed toward their plants. So much for plants. What about human beings? Are there any unbiased individuals who have had similar experiences with other persons?

You'd better believe it. The proponents of Silva Mind Control, for example, have discovered that by harnessing and focusing the powers of the mind toward persons who are in need, they are actually able to improve the physical and mental condition of those for whom they are praying. Oops! They do not call it "prayer," but is it not basically a similar spiritual power that they have uncovered?

The hard-line skeptics, of course, remain unconvinced. But the truly open-minded seekers of truth are at least amenable to the possibility that Christians are not so out-of-it as they once thought we were.

Most Christians take a ho-hum attitude toward all the research with plants and human potential movements and the like. They may not know *how* prayer works, but they do indeed know that it is effective.

Volumes have been written about prayer, but simple believers have known all along that Jesus was not kidding us. Prayer made in faith can move mountains.

Are Prayers Answered?

Do we get everything we pray for? Of course not. Our prayers are not always answered because we often pray for things that would not be good for us. God, in loving wisdom and wise love, does not give us something that would be harmful to us.

The situation is comparable to that of a child who always wants to eat candy and fast foods. A parent would be irresponsible to give a child too much of that kind of fare, even though the child wants it very much. When children grow up, they usually ask their parents more for things they really need. The parent tries to help because the things the children are asking for are good for them.

When we grow up spiritually and start asking for the right things to happen, then we find out that our prayer is always answered, too. It may not be answered in exactly the way we wanted it to be, but yes—the prayer is answered.

Praying for one another can be the highest form of service. Here we are not talking about just "saying our prayers," rattling off a lot of words that we memorized when we were younger. We are talking about tapping into the power of the Holy Spirit that is within us and directing the Spirit to those who need healing.

Time—that is the problem. We are too busy to pray. We are not too busy to party or watch television or go out to dinner, but we are too busy to pray. What we are really saying is that we do not perceive prayer as a real value. If it were genuinely important to us, we would find time for it. It is as simple as that.

Prayer requires commitment and belief. If we just give lip service to prayer and do not honestly consider it to be important, then our prayer will be weak and ineffective. But if we believe that our prayer works and if we give time to it, then the results can be stupendous.

Of those who do pray, many go about it only half-heartedly. That is another reason why their prayers are ineffective. They are simply not serious about it. A *life* of prayer takes discipline and concentration. It is like an art form or a dance or a sport. You must learn the rules. You must train. You must believe in your goal.

Once persons have become somewhat proficient at prayer, great things begin to happen. They are able to exploit the powers of mind and will, and work in cooperation with the Holy Spirit.

Is all this a lot of double-talk and mumbo jumbo? Not at all. Even science is finally coming around to the conclusion that during prayer something concrete and measurable actually happens. First of all, the one doing the praying is helped. Relaxing and healthful alpha waves are emitted by the brain during meditation. In addition, during deep prayer the endorphine system sends into the bloodstream a natural

substance that is chemically indistinguishable from a mor-
phine compound. So when some say that prayer makes them
feel better, they may be describing a physiological change that
is taking place.

Perhaps even more mind-boggling, science is now measuring physical changes that take place in other persons and
objects as a result of applied prayer.

Would it not be wonderful to use this God-given gift for the
benefit of your loved ones and our world so desperately in
need of healing? Our biggest obstacle is probably an inability
to believe that it is worthwhile. But I am sure about one thing: if
we ever get around to using this power, we can change the
world.

TURNINGS

The New Asceticism

Until recently, very few persons wanted to have anything to do with the "spiritual life." That was because being spiritual was frequently considered in opposition to being realistic.

Today the spiritual dimension is seen in the context of the whole person. Growing spiritually in no way implies a flight from one's body, from deep friendships, or from the real world. The key word in spirituality today is integration, not denial.

Years ago, the spiritual path often entailed beating down the body and repressing our subconscious drives. The idea was to fly up to some ethereal realm and turn our back on the world of the senses.

No modern author has dealt with this theme better than Hermann Hesse. The either/or, spirit/matter choice is a theme that runs through all his works. My favorite is his *Narcissus and Goldmund*. In this novel, two young monks have a parting of the ways. Goldmund leaves the monastery to find God in the marketplace. Narcissus chooses to look for God by spending his life in the monastery. As old men, the two are reunited and they share with each other what they have discovered. I shall not ruin the ending for you by revealing their conclusions.

This theme of choosing between matter and spirit makes no sense to contemporary persons. They yearn for a way to be whole and holy without turning their back on the world.

Does this mean that now it is easy to grow spiritually? No. One must pay a price to arrive at this sort of integration, just as one had to pay a price in years gone by. Purification and asceticism still have their place. It is just that the whole process today looks different because it involves a much more positive attitude toward the body and the mind.

In the past, asceticism included such practices as fasting,

wearing hair shirts, and sometimes even inflicting corporal punishment on oneself. Today's asceticism is much more positive: The athlete of the spirit eats properly, gets enough but not too much sleep, and exercises regularly. He or she reads every day, strives to eliminate fear, guilt, and anger, and tries to make love the basis of life.

Obviously one's motivation is extremely important here. If persons are watching their diet for the sake of vanity, or thinking positively so that they will make a million dollars, then the whole process has been subverted. The presumption here is that whatever is done in the new wholistic fashion is done to make the person more disposed to intimacy with God.

But is it all just an excuse? It seems so much easier to embrace this new wholistic spirituality than the old "beat the body into submission" form of asceticism. To that I say, "Just try it." The goal of the wholistic approach is to submit every aspect of our physical, mental, and spiritual self to the lordship of Jesus.

With the old asceticism it was far easier to delude yourself into thinking you were doing something great for the Lord. After all, not everyone sleeps on the floor or takes cold showers. But the new asceticism constantly calls us to purify every aspect of our lives. It never allows us to let up. The old asceticism produced saints: Catherine of Siena, John of the Cross, Teresa of Avila, and many others. It certainly has a proven track record. We do not know yet if the new asceticism will produce narcissists or saints. But we have to move on, trusting in the Spirit, with a spirituality based on our very best understanding of what a human being is.

Who Is Saving Whom?

Flirting with the living God is a dangerous undertaking. If we allow ourselves to be seduced, there is no telling how we may eventually end up.

Deep down we know this instinctively. That is why we cling

so desperately to the externals of religion. Then we are still in control. We are still able to "manage" God.

If, however, by the grace of God, we ever get a taste of that living reality that is the basis of religion, we know that we are in a whole new ball game. This new ball game has its own set of rules. And its own set of problems. One of the biggest problems with a genuine spiritual awakening is the possibility of encountering a strange experience called "inflation."

Spiritual inflation is caused by the inability to assimilate properly our newfound light and energy. What happens is that we are so overwhelmed by our encounter with the divine energies within that we start thinking we are on a par with the Creator.

In a certain sense, this is true. All the great religions of the world allude to participation in the divine nature. In the New Testament Jesus says, "Is it not written in your law, 'I have said, you are gods'?" (Jn. 10:34) Hinduism boldly asserts: "Thou Art That."

Good theology, however, insists on maintaining a distinction between Creator and created. Just as two lovers never lose their individuality, so we and God are not the same thing.

Neophytes of the Spirit are sometimes so overwhelmed by their religious experience that they fail to make this distinction. In their enthusiasm they want to tell everyone about their intense encounter with the Lord and sometimes act as if they themselves are the Messiah. The medium gets mixed up with the message.

A priest friend of mine says that anyone who has just had a religious experience ought to be locked up in a closet for six months. That is not a bad idea. In extreme cases the individual thinks that he or she is a kind of prophet or savior. In the most extreme cases, persons have to be institutionalized because of the ultimate delusion of grandeur: They think that they are God the Creator.

Never argue with or ridicule someone who has had a recent blast of spiritual energy. He or she will come down to earth soon enough. It will not take long for the person to discover that the conversion is incomplete, that Adam is alive and well, and that his or her own thorn in the flesh, whatever it might be, has not evaporated into thin air.

Is all this to say that we should not open ourselves to the living God? By no means. The alternative is absolutely depressing. Imagine living your whole life thinking that religion was nothing but a list of dos and don'ts! No thanks.

Take the plunge. Believe that you are a child of God and that God really speaks to you in your prayer and in your dreams and in a million other ways.

Take the plunge; you will be rewarded. You will learn that you are free, that you are loved unconditionally, that life has meaning, that you are precious in God's sight. By all means, do it.

Just remember that we are not the saviors; we are the ones who have been saved.

The Gift of Tears

No one can hope to have a sense of wholeness unless he or she is first of all broken.

Our lives are filled with the sin of pride. We refuse to submit ourselves to God. We insist instead on being in total control of our lives. We set ourselves up as the sole judge of all that is. It is the garden of Eden all over again.

Some individuals can perpetrate this deception almost indefinitely. They escape into the world of self-centered distractions and steadfastly deny their own creaturehood and sinfulness. Instead, they project their guilt onto others.

The trouble with this approach is that they cannot get away with it forever. Some of these individuals have nervous breakdowns, some become alcoholics or dependent on drugs, but most who hold out on God eventually just become mean, surly, miserable, moody, and aggressive.

All the while, God is seeking us out and calling us to our true selves, our personhood in Christ. If we are even the slightest bit open, God will eventually knock on our door so loudly that we will have to let him in. If we do, it will be the best move we have ever made.

This meeting with the living God is not all peaches and cream. In fact, it can be a soul-searing, painful experience, because we finally see ourselves as God sees us. All of our defenses fall, and our projections are burned away. We are convicted of our own sinfulness and confronted with God's love for us.

God's initiative may come suddenly and dramatically, like a dike bursting. Or we may be brought to new life slowly, like grass watered by a gentle spring rain. The circumstances leading to such a conversion opportunity are varied, but the effects are inevitably the same. When our conversion finally takes place, we weep—always on the inside, and very often on the outside as well.

This "gift of tears" signifies that the "former self," the false self, is dead. We no longer try to dominate others and project our guilt onto them. We are stripped naked before a living, loving God, and see ourselves as we really are. It is this contrast between God's goodness and our egotism that is the source of our sorrow.

Our tears are not all negative, however. We also shed tears of joy because we have discovered our true nature as children of God. We then understand that we have been reborn as offspring of the resurrection. We become aware of the divine spark within us and we are humbled and awed to consider that we have been divinized, called to share in the very life of the Trinity.

How important is it that we have this experience? The most important thing is that we somehow arrive at a state of brokenness so that the Lord can make us anew. The actual experience of weeping is not important in itself. It is the attitude behind the weeping that is crucial.

You say that you and God are getting along just fine, thank you, that you are keeping all of the commandments and the laws of the church, and that you see no need to admit your nothingness before him? Watch out! You may be deluding yourself.

A few Christians seem to have been in deep union with God all their lives. But most of us ordinary Christians have had to go through the painful process of conversion. Most of us instinctively recognize the importance of this "gift of tears" (at least its interior dimension); it is a body-soul statement of the simple truth of things.

Chances are you need to come to terms with your creatureliness. Has it happened yet? Only you and God know. But, for others, at least, one very good indication of true conversion has been the "gift of tears."

Religious Feelings

Many persons have the distinct impression that religion consists of rules and regulations, rituals and rip-offs. Consequently, if they ever penetrate behind this facade of religion and encounter the living God, they are thrown for a loop.

It is an almost overpowering experience to discover for oneself that the basics of one's religion are *true!* To be sure, they are presented in an imperfect way by imperfect teachers and writers, but the great religions of the world hold a real treasure within their earthen vessels.

When all of this dawns on a person during a religious experience, he or she frequently breaks down and cries, or wants to run and soar like an eagle. He or she wants to tell all the world about this moving experience.

Such an emotional "high" may last for several days, weeks, or months. The person is acutely conscious of walking with his or her Beloved. Personal prayer may occasion profuse tears of joy and love. But it is important to remember that those intense feelings of closeness to the Lord do not last forever.

When this happens, the person frequently experiences a sense of guilt. What did I do wrong? Why has the Lord left me? Such guilt is, of course, misplaced. Even though warm feelings are nice to have, and even though millions of persons have had undeniable religious experiences, we should never make the mistake of gauging our nearness to God by how close we happen to feel to him at any given moment.

There is an old saying in the spiritual life that the soul in trouble is very close to God. St. Teresa of Avila endlessly cautioned against attaching too much importance to religious feelings. She wanted her sisters to love God maturely—not to be tyrannized by fickle feelings.

Feelings are nice and probably necessary in the initial stages of spiritual growth. After all, without them how would we ever know for sure about God's power and love? But after God has proved his power and love to us, after he has cuddled us and fussed over us, he then wants us to step forth in faith.

Instead of accepting this stage of growth, many yearn for the good old days of tears and cuddly feelings. In fact, they may even become spiritual gourmands and rush out to devour the latest and most bizarre religious phenomenon they can find.

Religious feelings can be very illusory, whether we feel that God is our best friend or a million miles away from us. True religion is trusting in the person of Jesus and his central message that God loves us all unconditionally. It is letting that love of the Father take root in our hearts and overflow in love and justice to every man, woman, and child on planet Earth. It is believing in the fundamental goodness of life and all of God's creation.

Those who believe that religion is rules and regulations, rituals and rip-offs have obviously missed the point of what it is all about. But those who base their religion on feelings (either positive or negative) are equally mistaken. Christianity has always been about the white-hot, painful, life-giving fire of love that holds the universe together. To base it on anything else is a perversion of the religion of Jesus.

The Broken of Our World

The commercial says, "When you've got your health, you've got just about everything." This strikes a responsive chord in us and we all nod our heads in agreement. As an avid jogger and exerciser and health food eater and all that, I of course know the importance of maintaining good bodily health. When your body is in good shape, your mind and your spirit are affected, too.

But even good health can become a false idol. When we are feeling on top of the world, when we feel that we have everything under control it is easy to start thinking that we have outgrown our need for God. The same temptation is also present if we are very physically attractive, or very intelligent, or very wealthy.

That is one reason many persons in their twenties and thirties drift away from the Lord for a while. When you are in your physical prime, are at the peak of your mental powers, and have a few dollars in your pocket, you start asking yourself, ''Who needs God?'' The broken persons of the world are under no such illusions. When you are chronically sick or without a job or suddenly single again, it can sometimes turn out to be a blessing in disguise. Because then you know, you really know, that you do not have it all together and you need to rely on a power greater than yourself.

The broken persons of the world, the truly poor in spirit, are open to God in a way that the fortunate of the world will never be. That is why Jesus chose to associate, for the most part, with the rejects of his society. He hung around with the poor, the blind, the deaf, the lame, the lepers, the prostitutes, the outcasts. This of course offended the religious professionals of his day, just as similar behavior by Christians today continues to offend the self-righteous among us.

Jesus was not intentionally trying to offend anyone. He was simply choosing to minister to those who were open to what he had to offer. He knew he was not wasting his time with them.

Jesus could do nothing with the Pharisees. They were smug, arrogant, and full of pride. They were doing quite well without him, thank you. But were the Pharisees really happy? No one who lives a life based on anything but love can ever really be happy. It is just that some have always been a little better at fooling themselves and the rest of us into thinking they have it all together.

When you are working for your Rolls Royce, or your $250,000 house, or when you are sitting on top of the world, you can start kidding yourself that total human fulfillment is just around the corner. The poor in spirit, the broken of our world, know that they will never have any of these things. In that sense, maybe they are blessed. They have no one and nothing to turn to but God.

The soldier in the foxhole, the forty-year-old businessman on his back in the hospital after a heart attack, the paraplegic, the forgotten senior citizen, the down and out—they know deep in their hearts how fragile life is. They are only too aware that they are creatures, totally dependent on a power greater than themselves.

In that sense, maybe they are not really so unfortunate after all. The ones who are really in trouble are those who, for one reason or another, think they have outgrown their need for God.

Repression Is Regression

After a person has undergone a spiritual transformation, he or she may seem a totally different person. But not everyone who experiences a radical change in life has advanced spiritually. Sometimes a faulty understanding of spirituality actually causes a person to regress. He or she may *think* it is progress, but it may be nothing more than a buckling under to the superego (our set of childhood "tapes" telling us what we should and should not do).

How can we tell regression from progress? We examine a person's love level and freedom level. Is our experience of God one of love or one of fear? If we are experiencing an increase in self-acceptance and a growing love for the whole world, chances are that our experience has been a valid one. If we have just decided to "give in" to the God of a harsh moral code, however, we may just be regressing.

How about freedom? A true encounter with God should liberate us from an enslavement to a Ten Commandments mentality. Read the letters of St. Paul, especially his epistle to the Romans. He takes great pains to teach us that a person reborn in Christ is set free from the old law and is empowered to live by the new law of love.

For some reason, many Christians are not aware of this absolutely key teaching. You could drop Jesus and the Spirit from their religion, and not much would change. That is because they identify with the harsher aspects of the Old Testament God. When such Christians have a religious experience, it may in fact lead to repression of their personalities, based on fear and self-hate.

A very graphic portrait of religious repression is found in Flannery O'Connor's novel *Wise Blood*. The protagonist comes from an extremely strict, fundamentalist background. His unworthiness and sinfulness is drummed into him from earliest childhood.

As a young man, he totally rebels against this harsh God. In his rebellion, he throws out the baby with the bathwater. But at least he is trying to break his enslavement to the glorified superego masquerading as God. He decides to start his own church, the "Church Without Jesus Christ."

His very obsession with this harsh God, even in rebellion, indicates his lack of freedom. Eventually, his mania does him in. He completely breaks down and, as an indication of his "return to the Lord," engages in fierce penances. He blinds himself with lye, wraps barbed wire around his chest, and places sharp stones in his shoes.

Ostensibly, he has had some sort of "conversion" experience, but in reality he has simply abandoned his intuitions about the inherent worth of human beings. He has made no real progress at all. In fact, he was probably closer to the God of Jesus when he was questioning, doubting, and rebelling.

Repression is not progress. Repression is a sign of immaturity and seldom lasts very long. Almost inevitably the old repressed conflicts surface again, usually with devastating consequences.

The repressed, lobotomized personality may appear to be at peace. There are no more apparent questions, no more struggles. In reality, however, the person has chosen to be a vegetable instead of a thinking human being. In no way is that any kind of progress, spiritual or otherwise.

The glory of God is a person fully alive. Any fully alive person that I know of thinks, questions, struggles, wonders, gets angry, laughs, cries, cares, and shares. In other words, a fully alive person is like Jesus.

GROPINGS

Mystery of Life

I officiated at a baptism recently. It was a real pleasure to celebrate with so many persons the miracle of new life.

We placed the baby on the altar after the ceremony and stood around with lit candles symbolizing the light of Christ that was now burning within this new Christian. Intelligent, sophisticated individuals, all with tears of joy in their eyes because of the wonder of new life.

What is life? Put most simply, it is what happens to us between our birth and our death. It is a gift that none of us have earned. It is a mystery that none of us can adequately explain.

Sometimes I simply marvel at the gift of life. Why was I born in this country, at this point in history, surrounded and nurtured by this family and this set of friends? There are no adequate answers. There is only life—not a problem to be solved, but a mystery to be lived.

We see the intrinsic value of life when we observe the lifestyles of those who are battling to survive. The poor are involved in a harsh struggle for daily bread, for a roof over their heads, for heat in the cold of winter, for some human understanding (even if they try to reach such a state drugged with beer and wine). Their primary goal is make it until tomorrow.

Christians, too, solidly affirm the value of human life. Our tradition is one of outspoken defense of this marvelous gift since we see it as coming from the hands of God. Life for us is good in itself because it is a gift from God. It needs no further justification or legitimation. Our philosophy is in sharp contrast with that of some social scientists who speak of a "quality of life." They do not see life as being inherently good and worthwhile. They only value a life that is judged cosmetically beautiful or socially significant.

To such social scientists, a school for retarded children must seem to be a misguided waste of money and energy. After all, these children will probably never make any great contributions to the scientific community, nor are they likely to add to the Gross National Product. Some persons even question whether indeed these special children have any inherent right to life.

Students of history are quick to note that such rationalizations were at the basis of Hitler's plan for a "super race." The maimed and crippled were judged to be inferior. So were the Jews. Only the healthy, blue-eyed, blond members of the Aryan race were thought to be worthy of the gift of life.

We have not yet drifted quite that far in this country, but we are certainly on our way. Many persons see life as worthwhile only for the healthy, the intelligent, the cosmetically beautiful, the athletically fit. Little babies are a drag, retarded children are a cross, and the elderly are a burden. And so we legalize abortion, we fail to provide adequate funding for care of the mentally ill, and we treat our senior citizens disgracefully.

Somewhere along the line we have lost sight of what a beautiful gift life is in itself. Three cheers for Birthright, Right to Life, the Quakers, the Grey Panthers, the homes and schools for retarded children, and all other individuals and groups in this country that are standing up in defense of the inherent dignity of human life!

What Are You Accomplishing?

I had not seen my childhood friend for many years. We had played on the same baseball team and gone to the same dances. We had been close friends all through high school. But then I had entered the seminary, and we drifted apart. He never could figure what had gotten into my head to make me go off and study to become a priest.

He wanted to know if I was really happy. I assured him I had never been happier in my life. With an incredulous look on his face, he asked me a crushing question, "Tom, what do you think you are accomplishing? What do you have to show for your life?"

The answer of course is that, in terms of worldly accomplishments, I have not done very much and have relatively little of commercial value to show for my life. Yet I feel I am the luckiest man in the world. How is this possible? Quite simply, I refuse to measure the value of my life based on how much I have contributed to the Gross National Product.

Many persons who care about human beings have a rough time of it in American culture. We are all geared to measure a person's worth by worldly accomplishments. If a person has a fancy job title or has a lot of letters after his or her name, we are impressed. If the man or woman is not out there making money and doing something "meaningful," then the life in question is considered a waste.

On one occasion when I was giving a talk, I was asked to prepare a resume. "The audience will want to know about your credentials." So I wrote where I had gone to school and things I had "accomplished," and as I did so, I started to get a sick feeling in my stomach. I was thinking of myself as a marketable commodity. I felt the shallowness of letting myself be defined in terms of degrees and positions. None of those external criteria says anything about me as a person.

Our being impressed by worldly "accomplishments" is probably one of the reasons why those who live cloistered lives come under such a barrage of unfair criticism in the church. "What are they contributing to society? Isn't their life a cop-out, an escape?" There are many who do not understand that a peaceful life, lived in harmony with oneself, one's neighbor, and God, needs no further justification.

Contemplatives support themselves and pray for the needs of the world. It is not necessary for them to run for political office or work on Madison Avenue in order to make a real contribution to humankind.

The compulsion to justify ourselves based on "meaningful" accomplishments may be one of the reasons so many homemakers are being seduced by the call to do something "significant" in the eyes of others. What they are perhaps overlooking is the fact that being a good spouse and a sensitive, loving parent is no small task in itself, for a man or a woman.

One of the reasons for the weakening of family life is the inability of many men and women to look for happiness in their home lives. They are off seeking credentials and making "meaningful" contributions to society, often to the detriment of their marriages and their children.

The above thoughts are absolute heresy to proponents of the American dream. But, as a Christian, I choose not to buy into this aspect of our culture.

The drive for upward mobility, the compulsion to accomplish and succeed, is responsible for much of the unhappiness and suffering in our world today. As far as I am concerned, the only truly worthwhile accomplishment is living a graceful life before God and one's fellow human beings.

Spiritual Work

After celebrating Mass twice on a Sunday morning, I always feel absolutely drained. I have sometimes felt the same way after teaching a class or after leading a retreat or after a counseling session.

Wishing not to appear melodramatic, I would always keep my feelings to myself. Over the years, however, I have discovered a pattern. Practically every priest I know has reported similar experiences. They even use the exact same word to describe this feeling: drained.

What is going on here? How can only a couple hours of work so totally enervate healthy men? After looking into the matter, I have come to the conclusion that spiritual work is the hardest work of all.

At first glance, one would think that physical labor would be the most taxing. It is true that extensive use of the muscles can tire a person out. But most persons I know also report a physical "high" from a good workout. There is such a thing as a "good" feeling of tiredness.

Paradoxically, a good workout can actually energize a person. My mother says she will never be able to understand this. She thinks my father and his three sons and one daughter are a bit strange because we all feel "great" after a good workout. My dad simply loves to cut the grass, work in the garden, and shovel snow. All of us kids are physical-fitness fanatics. The more we exercise, the better we feel.

Mental work is much more draining than is physical work. After spending hours poring over facts and figures, businesspersons sometimes feel their head is ready to explode. Mental fatigue is something many of us have experienced. But mental work can also be exhilarating. New ideas and new insights are stimulating. When ideas come rushing forth in a spurt of creativity, a person is fortunate indeed. It is a peak experience that gives gusto to our lives.

Spiritual work, on the other hand, is very seldom so exhilarating. The one exception is when everyone in a group is more or less on the same spiritual wavelength. At times like that, everyone feels energized. Everyone is aware that the Spirit has clearly been at work.

More often, though, the spiritual facilitator experiences energy drain. That is because he or she is vulnerable, exposing his or her essence for all to see. There are some who are so spiritually hungry that they drain all the energy from the ones making themselves vulnerable.

There are two ways to deal with this energy drain. One is to just go through the motions. Read off the words, observe the rubrics, put everyone to sleep, and lead no one to the Spirit.

The authentic way I have found to gather more spiritual energy is to consciously plug into Christ so that one can use his energy. I am serious. Before I preach or teach or counsel or do anything else where my whole person is to be involved, I center myself and ask Christ to be my energy. The only time this prayer does not produce the desired results is when my ego

gets too much in the way and I start taking myself too seriously.
This insight, I think, can help any Christian. Whenever you
pray for anyone or anything, do it in the name of the Lord Jesus.
In that way it will be God's energy that is transmitted to others.
And perhaps some trace of it will stay with you.

Joy Amid Suffering

The worst part about going to any party is waiting for it to get
warmed up. For the first fifteen minutes or so, guests are
generally tense and ill at ease. The small talk is heavy and we
start wondering if we are in for a very long evening. Then, if we
are lucky, someone arrives who ignites the party.

Certain persons just have a way of turning any gathering
into an exciting event. We just know that after such a person
arrives, everyone is going to have a good time. I am not sure
what it is, but some persons just seem to have that magic
quality that enables them to lift us up when we are discouraged, or depressed, or lonely.

When we are feeling low, we can give such individuals a
phone call, and they lift our spirits right away. No matter
where we run into them, they are just naturally joyful and
graceful.

What is their secret? Why do these persons seem to be
immune from the problems that crush us? The truth of the
matter is, of course, that these individuals have the same
problems that we have. The difference is in how they handle
their problems. Their secret is that they see things differently.
Somehow they realize that in life the good far outweighs the
bad, that God is in control of things, and that in the end all will
be well.

It is not that such individuals are blind to reality, nor is it that
they have never suffered. It is just that they focus on the really
important things in life. They try to maintain the awareness that
they are children of God, brothers and sisters of Jesus Christ,
temples of the Holy Spirit, and members of Jesus' Mystical

Body. This is not a potpourri of pious platitudes; it is the truth about who we are.

Such an awareness ought to give Christians a different perspective on life. It should cause us to have a glint in our eye, a spring in our step, and a little smile always on our face. Not that life does not have its share of pain, of course. But, in view of God's friendship, our pain should not be the end of the world for us.

Giving in to our hardships may even be a subtle form of pride. It may indicate that we are taking ourselves too seriously. One of my favorite posters is of two little girls dressed up as clowns with mops on their heads. The inscription reads: "Don't take yourself too seriously." I have let that poster speak its message to me time and time again.

We should take God seriously, but not ourselves. If we remember that he is the master architect in life, then we can relax a bit and learn to enjoy life. When individuals insist on taking all of life's responsibilities on their shoulders, you have to wonder how strong their faith really is.

Balance is important here. It will do no good to slap each other on the back, wear a Pollyanna smile, and pretend we do not have any problems. This would only be a dishonest attempt to fool ourselves, and others would see right through it. We should have within us, however, an underlying peace and joy that no one can take away from us.

Our sojourn in life is really quite brief. Seventy years or so may seem a long time, but in the millions of years of evolution, it is just the proverbial drop in the bucket. We should do what we can to let some love move through our lives while we are here. And then let us put it all into God's hands.

Honesty Before God

Being a sinner is no obstacle to being a good member of the church. In fact it is a requirement. The church is the home of sinners. Those who claim they have no sin are liars. At least that is what St. John says. So if you are aware of your own brokenness and incompleteness, you are in luck.

Our sinfulness keeps us humble. It lets God be God. When we are aware of our own creatureliness, God can do something with us. That is why Jesus never got upset with anyone who was able to face his or her sinfulness. The only ones he lost his cool over were those who were self-righteous and considered themselves better than others.

If you try to fool God that way and pretend you have "got it all together," you are in big trouble. That is what the Pharisees of Jesus' time tried to do. The Pharisees were not evil people. St. Paul was a Pharisee. So were many of the religiously sincere persons of Jesus' time. Their mistake was in thinking that their scrupulous observance of the rules made them better than others. They were not aware of how insidiously infected they were with the sin of pride.

Like the poor, the Pharisees will be with us always. In fact, there is a bit of the Pharisee in each one of us. We fall victim to this mentality whenever we try to identify ourselves with all that is good and holy while trying to deny how really confused and scared we are at times.

We probably do this because we still think we have to earn our own salvation. We think we have to prove something to God and impress him by measuring up to all of the criteria for holiness. In so doing we forget that God's love for us is unconditional. No matter how crummy we might feel about ourselves, he is always gazing upon us with a smile.

Because his love for us is unconditional, we have nothing to fear in standing before him with utter honesty. Our fear stems from our inability to judge by any other standard than our own. Because we would find it difficult if not impossible to be so loving and forgiving with others, we automatically assume that God would treat us the same way. But Jesus tells us that just the opposite is the case. His God and our God is positively lavish in love and forgiveness. We can face our own sinfulness because we know that we have been washed clean by the blood of the Lamb. Our brokenness does not destroy us because we believe that when the Father looks at us, He sees only Christ.

The more God-conscious we become, the more we become aware of our own sinfulness. This is not some masochistic guilt feeling. It is just simply and humbly acknowledging the truth. A person slowly learns to accept himself or herself as a sinful human being.

The toughest step for human beings is admitting that they are in fact human beings. That is because we instinctively realize that, even though the truth will set us free, it will first make us miserable.

Just as "it isn't nice to fool Mother Nature," so it is not very smart to try to fool God. Our God does not want us to be plaster saints. He only wants us to face honestly the brokenness of our human condition. Only when we can finally admit that we are indeed earthen vessels can God do something with us.

Today Is All There Is

One of the rarest finds these days is a truly happy person. Everywhere you look you see sour expressions and downcast glances. Why does the world seem to be on such a universal "downer"? There are many reasons, obviously, but one of the greatest problems I find is the inability to live in the present.

So many persons are guiltridden over past failures and anxious about the future. They seem to be living everywhere except in the present. They are hamstrung to the point where life is passing them by.

For many years now, I have observed this inability to live in the present. In this respect, priests are much like everybody else. All through the seminary I saw young men who were afraid to be themselves, for fear they would never be ordained to the priesthood. Seminarians would suppress their true ideas and feelings because they were thinking of the future. "When I'm ordained I'll be a part of the system, and then I'll be able to get a lot more done."

That is what I heard for years. Now I see men who are ordained still repressing their ideas and feelings based on the same logic: "When I get to be a pastor of a larger parish, then I'll really be able to be effective. In the meantime it's probably best to play it cool."

I ask myself, what happens when the man becomes a prominent pastor? Does he then play it safe until he is a bishop? Will he make his move then, or is he going to wait until he is not just any bishop but the bishop of an important diocese? The waiting game seems to have no end.

Many of the laity play the same game. They are consequently just as unhappy and alienated from themselves as are their clerical counterparts.

First there is nursery school, then elementary school, preparing you for the great moment when you enter high school! But then you must plan ahead for college. Then graduate school, if you really want to make it big.

Yet, when you finally get out of the academic uphill scramble, it only takes one sales meeting to let you know that you are back in the same old system. When you make your quota, they give you a higher quota. You climb up and up, becoming vice-president or maybe even president of the company. Have you arrived yet? Not quite.

You must now look forward to that great American institution, *retirement*—when at last you will be able to enjoy life. But by that time your efforts to achieve and accomplish will have left you with a weak heart, fuzzy eyesight, false teeth, arthritis, sexual impotence, and an ulcer.

The only truly happy people I have come to know in my short life are those who have learned to welcome every new day as a gift from God. They are not depressed over past failures (what can you do about them anyway?), nor are they all worried about what the future holds in store for them.

Happy persons live each day as if it were their last. They take time to smell the roses, do not feel guilty about "wasting" time in conversation with friends, and, above all, have a great sense of humor. They can laugh at themselves. They are blessed with a faith in God. They know that, in the end, nothing human is worth getting an ulcer over. With God in charge, no matter what happens, all will be well.

Sometimes I am asked why I almost always have a smile on my face. It is almost as if some persons resent me for being so happy. A particularly joyful friend of mine has the same problem. She smiles so often that one of her six children woke her up one morning with the question, "What's the matter, Mommy? You weren't smiling!"

If some want to go through life as "angry young men or women" or "old grouches," that is their choice to make. But there is an honest-to-goodness alternative. Those who have discovered the marvelous art of living fully in the present have discovered one of life's best and most rewarding secrets.

Peaks, Plateaus, and Nadirs

A normal spiritual life has a combination of peaks, plateaus, and nadirs. In other words, we have our ups and downs, but usually we just keep on keeping on.

Some scholars say that the great religions of the world all grow out of peak experiences. Unless a person has some convincing religious breakthrough somewhere along the way, religion forever remains "out there," an account of what other, "holier" persons have experienced.

Religious peak experiences are valuable because they give a person first-hand, undeniable, experiential evidence of spiritual reality. They are problematic because some persons seem to be constitutionally incapable of such experiences. Persons who are obsessed with a need to control themselves, their environment, and others simply refuse to give themselves permission to "let go." Such individuals also find it difficult to laugh or to fall in love.

Most persons have at least one or two religious peak experiences in life in which they know that all is well with the universe. Such experiences can take place, for example, while climbing a mountain, walking by the seashore, or giving birth to a child. Such experiences can be enough to carry us through a lifetime.

But what about the nadirs, the dips and valleys of life? Such experiences also have spiritual value: They can help move us beyond our present lethargy. Carl Jung goes so far as to say that we should count ourselves fortunate when we are suffering from a neurosis. A neurosis serves to crack the husk of the ego and open us up to our higher self.

The highs and the lows are the fascinating times in our lives. We never forget them. I pray every day that I will never forget what it was like to be spiritually lost and then found by Christ. Such experiences serve as landmarks in life. They help us keep our bearings.

As fascinating as the highs and lows are, however, most of the time we move through life on a plateau. These times seem boring and uneventful, especially when we are always reading about the religious breakthroughs of other persons. The plateaus, however, are far from uneventful. During these times we get to consolidate our strength and to grow, quietly and undramatically.

We may not even think that we are growing at all. We feel as if we are on a treadmill and not making any progress. When others see us, however, they can see that subtle, yet real transformations have taken place in our personalities.

Some personalities (spontaneous individuals) seem to be more naturally open to peak experiences, some (introspective types) are often mired in the nadirs of life, while some (calm, low-key individuals) just coast along on their plateaus.

To put the whole thing in still another perspective, Jesus does not say that peaks, plateaus, and nadirs will be considered at all at the Last Judgment.

We do not have to worry if we are not having frequent religious peak experiences, nor should we be upset if we are sometimes down in the dumps. In the end, when we have to give an account of ourselves, the only thing that will ultimately matter is whether or not we have loved God and one another.

Dark Night

We have had far too much doom and gloom in the church. Any spirituality that helps us integrate our bodies and souls and find the presence of God in material things is certainly welcome. Writers like John Powell and Matthew Fox point out how much we are missing by being so negative about ourselves and the world.

As much as I enthusiastically agree with this much needed thrust in spirituality, however, I find that it is incomplete. Something is missing. Something vital. Any spirituality that ignores the pain involved in spiritual growth is less than totally honest.

To use only one example, consider the mid-life crisis. Author Gail Sheehy says most persons undergo it in their forties or later. The mid-life crisis is no fun. It is a time characterized by self-doubt, gnawing anxieties, nameless fears.

Some persons manage temporarily to escape it. Many become workaholics or alcoholics. They will finally have to face themselves on their deathbeds. But many others undergo a painful process of self-transformation, in which they finally accept themselves as weak, sinful, limited, and yet somehow worthwhile— even beautiful. For the religious person this may be accompanied by a fullblown "dark night of the soul." Certainly the "dark night" may happen at any age and at any stage of a person's spiritual journey. But, for some reason, it often strikes us around the middle of life when we are going through major life transitions and transformations.

This "dark night" is, without exaggeration, the most terrifying experience a person will ever undergo. One feels worthless, hypocritical, and rejected by God. It is, of course, the darkness before the dawn. It is a purification process leading one to a whole new understanding of oneself and God. The pain lies in the fact that the person feels out of control and does not have the slightest indication that there will ever be an end to the indescribable suffering and dread.

How does one manage to go through it or ever get out of it? By faith alone. Maybe the person has never really believed before. Now it becomes a matter of survival. You believe because you realize you are incapable of doing anything to save yourself. Only a loving presence will suffice. Not the god of the philosophers, but *Abba*, Father, the personal, intimate, loving God.

Jesus shows the way. By embracing our crucifixion as he did his—by submitting himself to the Father—we arrive at the peaceful eye of the hurricane. We then know experientially that we have been saved by a power greater than ourselves. There is no pride left, only humility. If our will to live is still strong, we realize that it has only been by the grace of God.

Minor crosses are a part of life, but a traumatic experience of this nature can be endured only once or twice in a lifetime. Its value is that it gives you religious certitude, humility, and a compassion so all-encompassing that you will never again be shocked by anything about yourself or anyone else.

I realize that all of this sounds terribly melodramatic and almost impossible to believe. When I went through my own dark night, I was totally shocked, because for thirty years of my life I had never even been depressed. In the midst of it, I was convinced that it was the worst thing that had ever happened to me. Now I see it as the best experience God ever gave me.

This is somber material, and not my favorite topic to write about. But I think it needs to be said. So, keep reading spiritual writers who point out the joys of Christianity. It is my own particular emphasis in preaching and writing, too. But be aware that authentic growth in the Spirit always has a price tag attached to it.

LOVE

Self-Love Is Not Selfish

One of the most misunderstood aspects of the spiritual journey is the role of self-love. Frequently we get the impression that self-love is the same thing as selfishness and self-indulgence. Nothing could be further from the truth.

A person cannot be mentally sound, let alone spiritually healthy, without a firm love of self. We love ourselves because we are a part of God's creation. We have a right to be here. We have been created little less than the angels. It makes no sense whatsoever to treat ourselves as little more than dogs.

The mix-up comes about when we confuse self-love with selfishness. Selfishness is ultimately self-destructive because it tries to maintain the illusion that the world revolves around the ego. The selfish person never thinks of the big plan. All he or she desires is the exaltation of the ego and personally pleasing sensations.

Self-love begins with the big picture. It tries to fit into reality instead of making reality fit into it. It loves God, nature, other persons, and oneself as a small but vital part of reality.

Persons who love themselves choose to be good to themselves. I often give the unsolicited advice "Be good to yourself." Almost invariably I get a strange look in return. We are geared to expect advice telling us to treat others well. We are not used to having permission to treat ourselves in an equally kind manner.

Whereas the selfish person is narcissistic, the person with true self-love is able to forgive and accept himself or herself. Two of the finest examples of those who had a healthy love for self are the Buddha and Jesus. Both took ample time to rest, to pray, and to spend time with friends. When Jesus said we are to love others *as* we love ourselves, he was giving us permission to give ourselves a break and be good to ourselves.

Apparently a lot of us have never absorbed that message. Even though Jesus did not have a Messiah complex, some others do. They drive themselves mercilessly and feel guilty if they are not constantly on the go and constantly giving of themselves. Others may admire them as hard workers and really dedicated parents, priests, or whatever, but they are to be pitied. Those who do not know how to relax are driven on by compulsiveness and a poor self-image.

Secure, healthy persons do not need any trophies. They know that they are loved by God and therefore have nothing whatever to prove. Their activity is conscious and comes from their love center.

The neurotically unselfish person is unhappy. It is written all over his or her face. Abraham Lincoln once told his secretary that he did not like the way a certain person looked. When his secretary reminded him that none of us can help what we look like, Lincoln responded, "After forty years of age *everyone* is responsible for what they look like."

Some neurotically unselfish persons are unhappy because they secretly resent what they are doing and they even resent the persons they are serving. Often they betray their true feelings by the way they look.

Active but centered persons, on the other hand, have an aura of peacefulness about them. No one is busier than Mother Teresa, but I have never seen a more peaceful face. It is obvious that she loves and accepts herself for what she is.

To push oneself unstintingly for others may be a subtle form of pride, a projection of selfishness. To love oneself properly is not selfish; it means to accept one's role, one's place, within the larger plan projected by God.

Perfectionism

One of the subtlest forms of self-hate is to demand perfection from ourselves. It is subtle because it may look very "spiritual" and noble; actually it is nothing more than an exercise in self-flagellation.

When we set up impossible, Godlike standards for ourselves, we are setting ourselves up for a colossal crash. It is a no-win situation in which we are virtually programming ourselves for anxiety, depression, and fatigue.

The sickness of perfectionism is something that frequently goes back to childhood. Many individuals had rigid, demanding parents who doled out their love only on condition that their child attain perfection. Because this never happened, the parents' praise was always conditioned with, "Next time try to do a little better."

Comedian Sam Levinson tells the story that his father was never satisfied with the grades he earned in school. One day young Sam proudly brought home a test on which he had received a grade of 95. His father's only comment was, "Who got the other five points?"

A lot of ministers and priests and sisters are infected with the sickness of perfectionism. Maybe it goes back to one of the most misunderstood lines of Scripture, "Be perfect as my heavenly Father is perfect." We have a lot of broken men and women in ministry, unable to accept themselves. The first rule of mental health is to accept yourself as you really are. You can never love anyone until you have a healthy love of your real self (not some idealized self).

One of the best schools of self-acceptance is, oddly enough, organized sports. When you compete in any organized sport, you soon learn that accomplishment is something relative. A .300 hitter in baseball is considered a blue-chip player. But a .300 hitter fails seven times out of ten. A fifty percent shooter in basketball is an all-star. But a fifty percent shooter misses half his shots. Babe Ruth hit 714 home runs in his career. But he also struck out over 1,400 times. He struck out twice as often as he hit a home run, but we look at his overall record and conclude that he did very well.

Persons in all walks of life need to recognize their human limitations. Sometimes you succeed and sometimes you do not. It is not a sin to fail at something. But by those infected with the sickness of perfectionism, failure is seen as a personal tragedy. Consequently, they may be so paralyzed by their own fear of failure that they never try anything innovative or creative. They may settle into the mob, the herd, of humanity and never learn to grow as a person.

The world and the church are never truly served by such mediocrity. The world moves forward toward Christ only when men and women dare to use fully their God-given gifts. Because our humanity is flawed, we will inevitably make our share of mistakes. But because we are also the Body of Christ, alive with the Spirit, beautiful things will happen, too. Those with a healthy self-image will praise God when they succeed and have a healthy laugh at themselves when they fail. The poor perfectionists, on the other hand, will be so afraid of others' impending criticism that they will cower in the corner of life and never launch themselves into the human-divine drama.

Perfectionists need our help. They secretly hate themselves and therefore cannot love others. If we can ever bring them the freeing, unconditional love of the Father, perhaps they will finally learn to accept themselves as the beautiful persons that they really are.

That Special Someone

It is generally recognized these days that healthy human relationships are necessary for one's spiritual growth.

It may seem strange to some that this is even an issue. But not too long ago, "particular friendships" were strongly discouraged in seminaries and convents. The implication was that somehow spiritual aspirants were expected to skip over human love and jump directly into a love relationship with God.

This, we are rightly told now, is humanly impossible. A human being must be nurtured in loving relationships as an infant and child; he or she must also be sustained by such relationships throughout life. We never outgrow our need to love and be loved.

Were those who discouraged particular friendships totally in error? Not really. They were trying in their own way to protect a very subtle, yet important, value in the spiritual journey. They were trying to call attention to the fact that human relationships can be an obstacle to spiritual growth.

Here is the way it works. The spiritual journey usually begins with a sense of loneliness and unhappiness. We sense in our hearts that something crucial is missing in our life. We know that we ourselves can never make ourselves happy. What will, in fact, eventually make us happy? We are not sure.

At this point many try to find their happiness through the acquisition of material possessions. But the fact of the matter is that you can be as rich as Howard Hughes or Daddy War-bucks, and yet not find your heart's desire. No material thing will ever satisfy the deepest longing of the human heart.

Most persons realize this fairly early in life. They sense that some form of authentic *personal* relationship is the only solution. But because the "God thing" either never happens to them or frightens them, some people figure that *human* relationships must be the whole answer.

Indeed, some human relationships are providential at this stage. If a person finds that "special someone" with whom one is compatible, it can be a great blessing.

Some individuals are compatible physically, mentally, and spiritually. They have what is known as a sacramental union; their union leads them to themselves, to one another, and to God.

Not everyone, however, is so fortunate. For them, the human relationship becomes an end in itself. God does not explicitly enter the picture. The human relationship becomes a *substitute* for one's relationship to God.

Perhaps this is what that old warning about particular friendships, so repulsive to us today, was trying to get at. It was a bizarre kind of warning that only God can ultimately satisfy the deepest needs of the human soul. In that sense, it was right on target.

No human being can be expected to enter into the soul of another. No human being can understand as God understands and love as God loves. To expect another to do so is to lay on that person a set of impossible expectations. It is virtually guaranteeing that the relationship will end in bitterness and unhappiness.

Once a person finds God, of course, then human relationships can become deeper and fuller than ever before imagined. Friendship between two persons who are rooted in the Lord must make the Father smile. Nothing could be more beautiful.

That "special someone" in our life can be a *revelation*—not only of himself or herself, but of God.

Pleasers

Our family loves to "discuss" things at the dinner table. We will discuss almost anything: the latest medical cure, the state of the economy, international relations, last night's television programs, local politics. With all of the heated exchange of opinions, we remain a very close family. Our secret? We respect one another's uniqueness.

This may sound like apple pie and motherhood, but it is nonetheless true. Many persons have never been given the psychological space in which to think or act for themselves. They are the "conformers," the "pleasers." Such individuals never fully grow up, no matter how much education or responsibility they have.

Psychotherapist Rev. Joseph Hart characterizes the "pleaser" this way: "Pleasers are persons who find their *significance*, their *value* as persons, in pleasing others; they do not feel significant unless they sense that they are pleasing others and that others like them. They fail to perceive their own dignity as individuals and strive to attain a mistaken dignity in a way that can never be satisfied."[1]

Of course there is a bit of the pleaser in all of us. All of us at times exchange pleasantries, observe polite social conventions, and try to be generally agreeable. The professional pleaser, on the other hand, is someone who derives his or her very significance as a person from pleasing others.

Pleasers are lonely and unhappy persons. They are lonely because they cannot express what they really feel for fear of alienating others. The pleaser is guaranteed unhappiness because, with these impossible standards, "failure" is a virtual certainty.

What the pleaser needs is an equal dose of humility and unconditional love. Humility gives us permission to be imperfect and make mistakes. Once we quit trying to play God, we can grow comfortable with the fact that no one ever has it all together. On any given issue we may be wrong. If we are wrong, it is not the end of the world. We are still "somebody," even though we may have made a mistake.

The greatest need of the pleaser, however, is for lots of unconditional love. Once we experience the unconditional love of the Father, we are free to drop all the masks and quit playing games. We then have an eternal identity that no one can ever take away from us. At last we are free to be ourselves. If someone disagrees with us on some particular point, we are not thrown for a loop. We still have our center.

Sometimes we experience this unconditional love of God through an explicitly religious experience. But more commonly we experience it from fellow humans. In any event, unconditional love can do wonders in helping us to become real persons.

It was because Jesus was so closely in touch with his Father's unconditional love that he was free to be himself. He answered questions the way he wanted to, and was not afraid to assert himself. In short, he did not live his life trying to meet other persons' expectations.

I mention the example of Jesus because many allow themselves to be treated like doormats as part of a sick religiosity.

He shows us that it is more important to be a real person than it is to spend our energy always trying to please others.

Notes
1. Bernard Bush, *Loneliness* (Whitinsville, Mass.: Affirmation Books, 1977), p. 45.

Working with Love

We do not work simply because we have to. It is part of human nature to use our brains and our hands to dig into the human enterprise. And why not? God so loved the world that he sent us his only Son. If the Father thinks the world to be so worthwhile, it is only natural that we too should take it seriously and immerse ourselves in it.

The Father did not create the world as a finished product. New things are happening all the time. It is our job to realize our dignity as God's cocreators and to love the world as does God. Our goal is to reflect back to the Father a grateful, loving, and just world.

All of this is good in theory but, unfortunately, many blue-collar workers find it hard to look at their work this way. They regard their jobs as a way to make money—no more, no less. Many factory workers consider their work boring, monotonous, and dehumanizing. They come to resent their work, even stooping to deliberate sabotage of products or machinery as a way of expressing their anger at the system.

Those who are somewhat better off and employed in relatively more meaningful work do not always understand why blue-collar workers are dissatisfied. After all, "they are getting paid for their work, and if they do not like it, they can always quit."

Yes, the workers can quit, but they hang in there because they love their families and they have bills to pay. You have to admire self-sacrificing individuals who love their families so much. But any sensitive individual has to be upset with a system that has persons spending one-third of their lives doing something they despise, just so they can continue to survive.

The church can help blue-collar workers in a number of ways. We can continue to support workers' rights to unionize and to demand decent working conditions. Any spirituality that sidesteps the need for this kind of social reform is unrealistic.

Having raised our voices in protest and having put our resources on the line, we can help in other ways. We can say and show more, much more, about the value of work done in love.

Hindus teach that a meal cooked without love is poison. The same applies to anything we do. If it is done with a spirit of resentment, it can sour our disposition and end up being counterproductive. It is not so much what we do that matters, but how we do it. Any action done out of love can be redemptive.

I think of Brother David Steindl-Rast, one of the real leaders in spiritual renewal in our country. When not on the road, he is known back at the monastery as "Brother Cook." He mentioned to a group of us that when he is preparing a meal for his brothers, he tries to do so with as much reverence as a priest saying Mass. Indeed, he said that for him his kitchen is his altar.

Consciously doing something out of love changes the nature of the activity entirely. Lately I have spent the final minute before saying Mass not thinking of my homily (as I used to do), but just loving the people in church. As Father John Powell says, performances never move hearts. Only love does.

What we do flows from what we are. We all need to support others who think and live in love. And we, as Christians, should keep in mind that when we do anything for others out of love, it is really Jesus Christ who, through us, reaches out and touches the world he loves so much.

CATHOLICISM

Why the Emptiness?

The spiritual renewal of externals in the Catholic Church envisioned by Vatican II is now largely in place. Practically all the innovations advocated by liturgical reformers of the 1960s have been implemented. We now have the liturgy in the vernacular. Laymen and laywomen are now involved as commentators and lectors. Offertory processions are the order of the day. The statues and gingerbread have been removed from the sanctuaries. Vestments have been updated and liturgical banners adorn the walls and the lectern.

But still a void remains. Inner peace and happiness still elude us.

The main reason liturgical renewal (along with the renewal of religious life and parish life) has fallen short of its goals is that we have made the mistake of identifying superficial, external changes with authentic, interior renewal. We fell into the trap of thinking that if we changed this gesture, or that program, or this rule, then we would somehow grow closer to God and be more true to ourselves. The gestures, programs, and rules are now updated, but many of us feel no closer to God than we did before.

This is not to downplay the great and beautiful changes that have taken place in the Catholic Church during the last twenty years. The revised way of celebrating the sacraments, for example, has brought great joy to many within the Catholic tradition. Baptism, the Eucharist, confirmation, matrimony, holy orders, and the anointing of the sick have all been very fittingly updated.

How many persons would prefer to return to the Latin liturgy? Not very many, I would guess.

We are generally pleased with most of the external changes

that have taken place, but the Lord continues to teach us the old lesson that he is not satisfied with external observances. Our programs, projects, and pet ideas have all too often become idols. We have frequently sought change for the sake of change, and in the process neglected the conversion of our hearts to Jesus. If we are not reborn in Christ in the depths of our hearts, then our external "accomplishments" are sheer folly.

Once again we are called upon to realize that busying ourselves with external changes—even institutional changes—is of no avail if it is not part of building an interior temple acceptable to the Lord.

Jesus' First Sermon

Jesus had a lot of time to prepare his first sermon. Not until he was thirty years of age was he baptized by John. Only then did he begin his public ministry. During all those hidden years, he had had a lot of time to think about his first sermon in his hometown, Nazareth.

It was a very simple sermon. He first of all unrolled the scroll of the prophet Isaiah to the following passage, which he read out: "The Spirit of the Lord is upon me; therefore, he has anointed me. He has sent me to bring glad tidings to the poor, to proclaim liberty to captives, recovery of sight to the blind, and release to prisoners; to announce a year of favor from the Lord" (Luke 4:18-19).

Then he rolled up the scroll again and handed it to the attendant, and sat down. Everyone was watching him. And then he preached the sermon: "Today this Scripture passage is fulfilled in your hearing." Apparently no one wrote down, or later remembered, what he said after that.

Jesus' first sermon was about bringing glad tidings to the poor, proclaiming release to prisoners. The church is supposed to continue the ministry of Jesus: to tell the spiritually and materially impoverished the good news about God's love and what it can do in their lives, to encourage them to believe in the power of love, to release them from bondage.

Does this sound like the church we know? Rather than set persons free, we have often crippled them with impossible burdens and then made them feel guilty when they were unable to carry those burdens.

We have—we *are*—a church that is still terribly unfree. We have a clergy who are generally as victimized as anyone else by all the shoulds and oughts and the impossible burden of trying to be perfect. The clergy are often in the same prison of self-rejection that cramps everyone else. It is good to remember the example of Jesus, who came joyfully to set captives free.

Christian Americans

The suburban community in which I am presently living is made up of Catholics, Jews, and Protestants. Some of the Jews—but not all of them—go to the synagogue on the Sabbath. And some of the Protestants and Catholics—but not all of them—attend church on Sundays. But apart from where they spend that one hour of formal worship each week, there is no noticeable difference in the way they go about living their lives.

According to recent sociological findings, suburbanites tend to live strictly according to the American values of economic success, upward mobility, health, status, rugged individualism, and the pursuit of pleasure.

If someone finds these values acceptable and feels comfortable with them, then that is his or her choice to make. The only point I want to make is that these values are not to be found in the New Testament. They are not Christian values. They have very little in common with the New Testament ethic of concern for one's neighbor, meekness, personal poverty, and a communitarian sharing of one's possessions, as preached by Jesus.

There was a time when Catholics tended to identify

themselves more by their religious affiliation than by their nationality. We called ourselves "American Catholics." It is my contention that the emphasis has changed completely; now we consider ourselves to be "Catholic Americans." The change has been subtle, but it is potentially lethal.

According to the secular values of the culture in which we live, the greatest person is the one who is served by others. The great person is the one who is admired for his or her accomplishments, status, and power.

Jesus turned the world's value system completely upside down by teaching us that the greatest in the kingdom of heaven is the one who serves his or her neighbor. We cannot subscribe to the values preached by the leaders of this world. We must be different. We must be willing to wash each other's feet.

This teaching of Jesus goes over like a lead balloon these days, especially in the suburbs. It seems to go against all the Horatio Alger principles we were taught as children. Many suburbanites have worked quite hard to get what they have, and the last thing they want to hear is the invitation to share more of their wordly goods with those who are less fortunate than they are.

We already have enough guilt to last us a lifetime, and so it would suit us better to dispense with this somewhat awkward and unAmerican aspect of Jesus' teachings. But if we are to be authentic to the whole gospel, then we do not have the luxury of choosing those aspects of it that happen to fit into our own particular value system. The message of Jesus must be preached and lived in its entirety.

This meditation is somewhat embarrassing for me to write because I have to struggle as much as anyone else with the question of how to be both a Christian and an American. Priests go to the same schools, listen to the same Fourth of July speeches, and read the same books as everyone else in this country. It is just as difficult for us priests, with our comforts and middle-class lifestyles, to hear the message that maybe the American way is not the lifestyle that Jesus envisioned for his followers.

I am not promoting guilt, but it seems to me that many of our values are more American than Christian, and this frightens me.

Nice and . . . *Unchallenging*

We live in a nice country and worship in a nice church made up of a lot of very nice persons. But Jesus was not nice at all. He was challenging, confrontational, unorthodox, paradoxical, radical, prayerful. He was all of these things and more. No one ever called him nice.

The early Christians were not nice either. They broke away from traditional Judaism, refused to bear arms, and literally went underground. But somewhere along the way we became awfully nice. In fact, Christianity today is specifically aimed at turning out nice persons.

The church should always have as one of its primary goals to give comfort to people. But a goal of at least equal importance is challenging people to grow more and more in the Spirit of Christ. When everyone is worried about being nice, no one grows.

We Catholic Christians are no longer at the cutting edge of our society's spiritual growth. We discovered a long time ago that nice persons and nice institutions are rewarded, and those that call for change are disliked and systematically ignored.

We are often afraid to challenge one another. Nice priests give nice sermons, everybody feels good, and the priest is considered a nice guy. In the process, we all become mediocre and trite.

Growing in the truth is always painful. Artists in particular suffer much; they are seldom nice persons. Artists refuse to let us get comfortable. They make us face our present truth and challenge us to move courageously into the future. Consequently, real artists are seldom recognized while they are alive. They must take a back seat to the hacks who narcotize us with an idyllic, idealized, false picture of who we are.

One would hope that the church would be a little more courageous in calling us and our world to get on with life as Christ called us to live it. But the church is us, and we are weak, and we are afraid to rock the boat. We want to be truthful, but we are also afraid to ruffle anyone's feathers.

Thank God some in our midst have extricated themselves from this mediocrity. In fact the Catholic Church has an all-star cast of saints and mystics and spiritual giants who have seldom been nice but have always been real. Francis of Assisi, Ignatius of Loyola, Catherine of Siena, Teresa of Avila, John of the Cross, Thomas Merton, Maximilian Kolbe, Dorothy Day, Mother Teresa. The list goes on and on.

We can be justifiably proud of those individuals, but I do not imagine that any of them appreciates being put on a pedestal. Christianity is not a spectator sport, nor is it intended for a spiritual elite. Our church has produced some incredibly genuine human beings, but the silent majority seems mired in mediocrity.

Maybe it is expecting too much to hope that we can once again become the spiritual cutting edge of our world. Maybe it is unrealistic to expect that the majority of the Catholic community will one day try living out the faith rather than just talking about it. But one thing is certain: Jesus wants us not to be nice, but to be real.

Used to Be

Everywhere you go these days, you run into persons who used to be one thing or another. I used to be married. I used to be a priest. I used to be a charismatic. I used to be in Cursillo. I used to be in Marriage Encounter. I used to be a Catholic.

Our age is one of constant flux. Everyone is on the move, if not from one part of the country to another, then from one involvement to another. This is not just a hard time for lovers; it is a hard time for many to commit themselves to anything.

This kind of shift in loyalties is not all bad. Authentic growth necessitates change. Those who settle back into their comfortable securities may just be shying away from the challenge to grow. The temptation to smugness is always there. Consequently the tendency not to absolutize any movement or any walk of life can be a sign of growing authenticity in modern society.

But obviously all of this has its limits. For example, I find it somewhat puzzling when I meet persons who claim they used to be Catholic. Catholic means "universal." There should be room in our church for everyone. Our religion is designed to be inclusive, not exclusive. If any idea is true, it should eventually be incorporated into the collective wisdom of Catholic tradition.

The process admittedly is a slow one. The church thinks in terms of centuries, not hours. The problem with this is that most of us are not planning on being around for centuries. We walk across life's stage for one brief moment and we would like everything to be changed yesterday.

When change does not come according to our time schedule, we move elsewhere. If we embrace one of the other great religions of the world, it would not be so bad. Those religions are also sources of God's authentic revelation. But I have two problems with this approach. First of all, those religions do think in terms of centuries. Secondly, according to Dr. Takeo Doi of the University of Tokyo, it is psychologically dangerous for those with a Western mind-set to immerse themselves in Eastern religions.

So now what? We may take an eclectic approach. We select some of the various crash courses in instant enlightenment. We sample a smorgasbord of human potential psycho-technologies and assume that by running off to study TM or yoga or rolfing or EST or any one of a variety of other costly courses, we are finally going to get it all together. But frequently in the end we are more mixed up than when we began. The wisest course of action may be to return to our religious heritage.

Much of this searching takes place as we approach middle

age (thirty-five or so). Psychologist Carl Jung said middle age was such an important time in a person's life that there should be schools for the middle-aged. Then it dawned on him that we already have such schools: the great religions of the world. If we can plumb their depths, we will arrive at mental and spiritual health.

Admittedly, at first glance, it may not look as if our churches are capable of satisfying modern society's spiritual hunger. We seem fixed on regulations and structures. If these things are an end in themselves, they are bad. If they are to protect spiritual experience, however, they have their place. The trick is to cut through the externals so that we can get to the deeper truth of our religion. The truth is definitely there. It just takes a bit of creativity to find it.

Once we can tap the marvelous truth of the Catholic faith, we are free. We are rooted. We are saved from the anxiety and panic and dread of a meaningless existence. Then and only then, we have the psychological and spiritual security to incorporate the good that is found in today's various human potential movements.

Can You Say "Praise the Lord"?

Can you adequately explain to someone the feelings that you have for your best friend? Can you describe in words what you felt when your first child was born? Probably not. Certain experiences are meant to be appreciated, not explained.

That is essentially the way members of the Charismatic Renewal movement feel about how they experience and express their faith.

For so many years we were *taught* our religion. It was basically an intellectual experience. If you received high marks in religion, it meant that you had memorized the answers in the Baltimore Catechism. A boy may have been a real troublemaker, but if he knew the correct answers he received good grades in religion class.

During those years we learned all about Jesus Christ; our approach to him was very intellectual. We knew Jesus in the same sense we knew the pope or the president. We knew and appreciated what he had done, but most of us did not experience Jesus as a living reality.

For many Christians, this spiritual void has been filled by what is called Charismatic Renewal. The charismatic movement is based on the assumption that many adult Christians have never actually made a firm decision to turn their lives over completely to the Lord. When this decision is made, not just on an intellectual level but by a response of the total person, there is frequently experienced a feeling of closeness to Jesus that could never before have been imagined.

The person who experiences this "baptism of the Holy Spirit" feels reborn to a new life and frequently wants to shout about his or her conversion from the nearest rooftop. It is this initial zeal that causes some pentecostals (another name used for members of the Charismatic Renewal movement) sometimes to come across as being a bit pushy. It is the last thing in the world that they want to have happen, but their joy and enthusiasm actually frighten off some other Christians.

I have problems with some of the very literal interpretations given to particular passages of Scripture by charismatic followers, but I am convinced that the main thrust of the movement is sound and true. The American bishops have encouraged the Charismatic Renewal movement; they believe it is an authentic work of the Holy Spirit.

How does all this fit into the Catholic tradition? After all, Catholics do not clap their hands and shout "Praise the Lord!" while someone is preaching a sermon or leading a prayer session.

Well, the whole thing gave me a queasy feeling in the pit of my stomach when I first heard about it, I must admit. But attending a Charismatic Renewal convention made a believer out of me. Eight thousand persons were walking around the city bursting with joy at the love of Christ they were personally experiencing.

There were some kooks at the convention, of course, but the great majority of the participants seemed very well-adjusted and balanced. They were full of joy. And that is not the kind of thing you can fake. Charismatics are on to something real; it is producing genuinely good results in their lives.

There are many paths that lead to the Lord. The Charismatic Renewal movement is only one of them. If you are satisfied with your relationship with the Lord, then by all means keep on with what you are doing. But if your spiritual life has become arid, maybe you should look into what the charismatics have to offer.

They have made a believer out of me, cautious and skeptical as I am.

Words Are Like Fingers

Words are important, but they are no substitute for experience. I pity those persons who are so fascinated with words that they never really get around to living life to the full.

Wars have been waged and schisms have developed over words. That is because some persons begin to identify a given word with the reality it stands for. They think that if you change the word, you change the reality.

We Catholics, as much as anyone else and more than some others, used to get all hung up on words. I thank God for Pope John XXIII who told the bishops of Vatican II that our faith is one thing and how we express that faith is something else entirely. An experience is far more important than its verbal formulation or articulation.

When some parts of the mass were translated into English, for example, many Catholics simply could not adjust. They took solace in the fact that at least the words of consecration were still in Latin. But when the *Hoc est enim corpus meum* was changed into "This is my body," many simply could not handle it. Changing the words was like changing the reality.

Those who really experience God in prayer realize that we

cannot capture God in a neat little box. We cannot name him, or adequately describe him. Even the word "him" is inadequate. As Pope John Paul I told us, "God is as much our Mother as our Father."

At first glance, this seems like a real problem. We do not seem able to have the final word with God. Actually, this is one of the most providential aspects of our life.

If Christians or Hindus or Buddhists were absolutely sure they had the final word, they would probably start "holy wars" all over again. But because "no one has ever seen God" (John 1:18), we are much more respectful toward one another.

This is in no way to relativize Christ. He is the final Word. It is just that we are not sure we have fully grasped this final Word. He eludes our definitions and our categories. Our understanding of Christ is necessarily conditioned by our culture. Paul understood Christ in one way, Augustine in another, Thomas Aquinas in another, Teresa of Avila in another. Which one was right? They were all right—but none of them had the whole truth. They understood him as best they could, but they never *fully* understood him. That is because we can speak about Christ only with our human words, which are always inadequate.

Buddhists have a saying that words are like a finger pointing to the moon. If you want to see the moon, do not get too attached to the finger. Do not be too attached to words. Look beyond words for the reality to which they point.

One of the greatest examples in our tradition of someone who never got her finger in the way of her vision was Teresa of Avila. We now read her works, which all came out of her personal experience, as spiritual classics. But they were not recognized as classics when they were written. In fact, they were put in writing at the request of her confessor who had doubts about her orthodoxy. Teresa trusted her own experience and was not particularly worried that the way she expressed herself was unique.

We, like Teresa, are being asked by the Holy Spirit to look out into the night in faith and not cling to our old formulations and our comfortable securities. This is an age made for explorers, not settlers. God's love is constant, the victory of Christ assured, and the presence of the Holy Spirit a reality. That should be enough for men and women of faith as we venture forth into the twenty-first century.

EXAMPLES

The Spunky Ones

Most universities find it difficult to raise money. But when Fordham University wanted to build an enormous fieldhouse, officials raised all the money they needed overnight. What was the secret? They named it after one of their most famous alumni, the late Vince Lombardi.

Lombardi, the former coach of the Green Bay Packers, was an aggressive, no-nonsense kind of person. He has immense appeal among the movers and shakers of our society who buy his philosophy of hard work and discipline. Naming the fieldhouse after him was a stroke of genius. Donors lined up to give their money as a way of endorsing his philosophy.

I personally have no trouble with aggressiveness and competition. I have been playing in organized sports since I was eight years old. But aggressiveness has its limits.

Father Matthew Fox rightly points out that when we are growing up we hear a lot more about competition and aggressiveness than we do about compassion. Compassion is a gospel value. No one can be too compassionate. But an overly aggressive person can be destructive.

How do we strike a balance between being spineless and being pushy? It seems to me that our aggressiveness, to be a gospel value, must be sensitive, patient, and prayerful.

Being sensitive does not mean letting others kick us around. The ethnic groups in our country would still be living near the Statue of Liberty if persons had not had the gumption to move out and take a risk. But in moving ahead we must always be sensitive to others, too. Sometimes charity demands a compromise, at least with our own timetable.

Aggressiveness must, therefore, also be patient. If I am sure I am right, I can afford to wait. Patience is a sign of strength. In fact, the stronger a person is, the less he or she needs to *show* strength.

But the most important test of our aggressiveness is whether or not it springs from spiritual motives. The "old man" dies very slowly. Our egocentric self is always ready to rear its ugly head. It is the easiest thing in the world to be aggressive for egocentric purposes. Am I pushing for some idea because I have prayed about it and honestly believe it comes from God, or is it just some scheme to enhance my false self? Dom Maruca, a Jesuit spiritual director, says that he refuses to discuss any serious problem with the priests and sisters who come to him for help unless they have first of all prayed over the problem. There is a lot of wisdom to this approach.

But once we feel reasonably confident that our idea or insight is from God, we should push for it, sensitively and patiently.

Teresa of Avila felt that God wanted her to begin a reformed order of Carmelites. Her efforts were initially rebuffed by the regular Carmelites. But she secretly went ahead with the building of her new convent. That was how confident she was. But she was also sensitive and patient. It took her twenty years before she eventually was able to bring her plan to fruition.

Thomas Merton felt that he was called to live apart from the rest of the monks in his monastery. At first he was rebuffed, but he kept sensitively and patiently coming back to his superiors. Eventually, after many years, he was able to build his cabin in the woods.

The Vince Lombardi philosophy—"Winning isn't everything, it's the only thing"—leaves me cold. It is too susceptible to the interference of the ego.

But three cheers to the "spunky ones" of our world and our church, as George Washington Carver used to call them. Many persons stand on the sidelines of life and cynically complain about things. The "spunky ones" have the courage to dream dreams and are willing to pay the price to see their dreams realized.

Well-Adjusted

A sure way to strike terror in the hearts of parents is to tell them that their child is not "well-adjusted." In this country, in particular, we seem to regard "adjustment" as one of our supreme national values. But, as Morton Kelsey asks, what if the group or idea or lifestyle to be conformed to is defective? What good is it adjusting oneself to a particular group if the group badly needs help?

It seems to me that making a fetish out of "adjustment" is a sure way to encourage mediocrity. Greatness in any form is usually accomplished by persons who are a little bit different from the rest of the herd.

Albert Einstein was always considered a "weirdo." When he went up to receive his Nobel Prize he wore a tuxedo. But he had forgotten to wear socks or tie his shoes. Was he "well-adjusted"?

When we think about famous artists and writers, it is difficult to find a "well-adjusted" one among the group. Ernest Hemingway, William Faulkner, Paul Cézanne, James Joyce, Andy Warhol, Edgar Allan Poe, and many others have all been characterized as eccentric or worse. But what an incredible contribution these "maladjusted" persons have made to our self-understanding!

In the ways of the Spirit, too, greatness has usually been accomplished by persons who were considered a bit strange. The saints and mystics were not the type to conform to established ideas and lifestyles. They were the visionaries who pursued the inner call no matter what others happened to think of them.

Psychologically speaking, it is crucial to separate oneself from the herd and be true to one's belief. Thomas Merton said, "The mother of all lies is the lie we persist in telling about ourselves. And since we are not brazen enough liars to make ourselves believe our own lie individually, we pool all our lies together and believe them because they have become the big lie uttered by the *vox populi,* and this kind of lie we accept as ultimate truth."[1] The big lie would have us believe that society is fine just as it is. To be a spiritual person, then, would be to ratify the values of society and not make any waves. Because the big lie is so seductively attractive, only the spiritually strong are capable of resisting it. But the strong who do resist must be willing to pay the inevitable price of crucifixion at the hands of the mob.

Thank God for all those spiritual giants who were strong enough to be true to their own convictions. As far as I can see, none of our saints was a conformist. But where would the church be today if:

- Benedict had not founded a religious community?
- Bernard of Clairvaux had not shown the union of divine and human love?
- Thomas Aquinas had not shown the compatibility of philosophy and theology?
- Francis had not called the church to a simpler lifestyle?
- Catherine of Siena had not called for the reform of the papacy?
- Teresa of Avila had not dared to take the inner journey seriously?
- Ignatius had not cultivated Catholic intellectuals?
- Thomas Merton had not shown the compatibility of Christianity and Eastern religions?
- Teilhard de Chardin had not shown the compatibility of evolution and Christianity?
- Pope John XXIII (against the advice of his advisors) had not summoned the Second Vatican Council?
- Mother Teresa had not left her traditional religious order to found a new group of sisters dedicated to working with the destitute?

It should also be added here that nonconformists must pay the price of being misunderstood and ridiculed. Each of the giants listed above suffered greatly for his or her contributions. But none of them settled for mediocrity.

This is not to imply that every "maladjusted" individual in our society or in our church has achieved greatness. But it is to say that greatness of any magnitude is seldom accomplished by those whom society calls "well-adjusted."

Notes

1. Thomas Merton, *Conjectures of a Guilty Bystander* (New York: Doubleday and Co., 1966), p. 71.

Sacristan Saint

His name was Franz Jaegerstaetter. Chances are you have never heard of him. But many consider him to be a modern saint.

The reason why he is not very well known is that his lifestyle is an indictment of the church in Germany and Austria during World War II. Many of those most threatened by his courage, especially priests and the hierarchy of the church, become very nervous whenever his name is mentioned.

Franz was a full-time church worker in a little town in Austria. He was a sacristan. His job was to help the priests prepare for the celebration of church ceremonies. He was married and the father of three daughters. There was not much special about him except that he was one of those rare individuals with courage and firm principles.

When Austria voted on whether to join the Third Reich, Franz was the only person in his village who cast a dissenting vote. No display of fireworks—just a simple man with the courage of his convictions.

But then Franz was drafted into the German army. There was no way in good conscience he could participate in what he prayerfully concluded was an unjust war. So he decided he would not go.

Everyone then tried to reason with him. After all, the church had taken no public stand against Hitler. So who did he think he was anyway? All of his friends and neighbors tried to talk some sense into him. His mother tried. So did his employer. So did the friendly parish priest. "Franz, Franz, you are only a simple sacristan. Our church leaders have welcomed the alliance. Why be so arrogant? And what about your wife and beautiful daughters? Who will take care of them?''

Franz decided to seek the advice of his local bishop. Unhappily, he received the same advice: Don't make waves.

Being a loyal son of the church, however, Franz was a man of conscience. So he went to prison. While Franz was imprisoned, the Catholic chaplain made one last attempt to talk some sense into him, but all to no avail. He was tried in Berlin and beheaded as a traitor in August 1943.

His ignominious death was one of the few bright spots in an otherwise sad performance by the church. But today there is a movement in support of his canonization. The main spokesman for his cause is, poignantly enough, the Catholic prison chaplain who tried to talk him into ''cooperating.''

Admirers visit his burial site. There has been a documentary about his life on Austrian television. A stained-glass window has been designed in his honor. His name was publicly mentioned during the Second Vatican Council. The people from his village still think he ''went a bit too far.''

Franz Jaegerstaetter is an example of someone who lived by the law of love. Seeing his example, we can praise God for Franz's life rather than let ourselves be depressed by the wholesale failure of the church in Nazi Germany and Austria to preach the gospel in season and out of season.

Institutions usually seek to protect their own interests. That is just the way human nature operates. And the church is a human institution—but it is more. It is made up of real persons, many of them heroic, many of them truly Spirit-filled. Persons such as Franz made us all aware that in our earthen vessels we carry a real treasure.

Prophetic Troublemakers

Have you ever wondered to yourself what could possibly be going through the minds of those who spark dissent within the church? After all, as the Body of Christ we should learn to work together harmoniously. Does not dissent cause internal strife and scandalize those outside the church?

As difficult as it is for most of us to understand, prophetic figures who point out the things that are wrong in the church have their part to play too. In fact, St. Paul considers prophecy to be the best of the charisms in the early church. (See 1 Cor. 14:1.)

The history of prophecy is long and stormy. In the Old Testament the prophets tried to discern God's working in historical events. This often meant denouncing rulers whenever they were violating their obligations to God. Because the rulers did not particularly care to be confronted with their shortcomings, they usually had the prophet put to death.

Although Jesus of Nazareth defies ultimate categorization, he is, according to Scripture scholar John L. McKenzie, more like a prophet than a priest. His style was one of confrontation. The prophetic style of Jesus grated on the nerves of the religious leaders of his day. He was considered a dissenter, a troublemaker.

Time and time again in the two-thousand-year history of the church, the pattern has repeated itself. Charismatic, prophetic figures have arisen, only to be rejected by the established leaders of the day.

For example, St. Benedict was hated by rival monasteries for his "new way." St. Peter Celestine was hounded from the Vatican because he wanted to institute needed reforms in the papacy. St. Francis of Assisi was considered to be a "kook," St. Catherine of Siena was judged "arrogant," St. John of the Cross was beaten up by the members of his own monastery, and St. Teresa of Avila was written off as a "neurotic."

What did all these saints have in common? They had new ideas that were a threat to the status quo. They were troublemakers. All had to pay a price—rejection and sometimes death. *Later* everyone praised them for their courage and foresight. The church canonized them and today everyone testifies to their greatness. But not while they were alive.

Prophets hope that history will render them a favorable verdict. But they are wise enough to know they cannot expect much support from their contemporaries.

Are there any recent examples of this pattern? Take the case of John Courtney Murray, the theologian from the Catholic University of America. Because of his "controversial" ideas on religious freedom in the 1950s, he was banned from teaching and lecturing at the university. But as it turned out, he eventually became the principal draftsman for the Declaration on Religious Freedom issued by Vatican II.

He and other reformers have two qualities in common: loyalty to the church and a sense of humor. Even when they are misunderstood, their love of the church is not diminished. In fact true prophets criticize the church because they see that it can be improved. They point out its blemishes because they recognize it as the Bride of Christ.

A good sense of humor is also important. True prophets refuse to take themselves too seriously. They are in no way self-righteous. They realize that neither the church nor the world rests on their shoulders.

Most of us are not called to be prophets. But inasmuch as there is a scriptural and theological and historical basis for such a role in the church, we should at least consider the possibility that "dissenters" may be unrecognized prophets. Disagreement is not necessarily a proof of disloyalty.

Modern Heroes

Believe it or not, there are still some individuals in the twentieth century who value their principles more than their personal comfort.

Columnist Claude Lewis of the former *Philadelphia Bulletin* once wrote about three modern American heroes who can serve as an inspiration to us all. The three men have widely divergent backgrounds. One is a baseball player, one a government bureaucrat, and one a federal judge.

The "capital sin" that all three committed was that they told the truth and bucked the system. Most of us, instead, live by

the specious advice, "If you want to get along, go along."
These three men refused to go along. Consequently, of course,
they had to undergo a lot of suffering. Anyone who insists on
speaking the truth knows that suffering is the inevitable price of
personal integrity.

The baseball player was Curt Flood. He sued professional
baseball over the "reserve" clause back in 1969. He reasoned
that it was unjust that a baseball team could "own" a player.
Flood left his team, singlehandedly fought nineteen mil-
lionaire owners, lost a year's salary in legal fees, and was not
publicly supported by a single major leaguer. He won his case
in court and today, while not personally any better off, at least
has the satisfaction of seeing many others benefit from his
courageous stand.

Of course, many people today feel that the pendulum has
swung too far in the other direction and that the players are
now the ones exploiting the sport. That may well be the case,
but, when Flood played baseball, the owners were clearly
taking unfair advantage of the players. Curt Flood was the first
one and, at the time, the only one to have the courage to put
his career on the line in defense of a principle.

The government bureaucrat was A. Ernest Fitzgerald of the
Pentagon. He too made the mistake of telling the truth. He
informed Congress about a $2 billion overrun on a govern-
ment project. His job was "eliminated" suddenly, and he
fought in court for years to get it back.

The federal judge was Frank M. Johnson, Jr., of Alabama.
He was the one responsible for the full integration of
Montgomery's public transportation. Johnson has been under
armed guard for over twenty years. His son committed suicide, explaining that no one had any idea what it was like
living in Alabama and being the son of Frank Johnson.

There are indeed heroic men and women around these
days. Even the church has its share. One who immediately
comes to my mind is Pierre Teilhard de Chardin, a French
Jesuit who died in the early 1960s.

Teilhard was a scientist as well as a priest. He saw no

contradiction in being both. His superiors saw otherwise. Because of his "dangerous" ideas he was subjected to some of the most inhumane treatment that one could imagine.

First, he was forbidden to accept a chair at the University of Paris. He was then sent to China, to get him out of Europe. When he eventually returned to Paris, he was immediately sent out of the country again, this time to the United States.

While in the United States he was forbidden to lecture or publish. In fact, his superiors never permitted him to publish any of his books or articles during his lifetime.

The week before he died, at the age of seventy-four, he asked himself whether he had been deluding himself during his entire life. After all, he reasoned, how could he alone be right and all of his fellow Jesuits wrong? He died a broken man. At his funeral only a handful of personal friends were present. The final indignity was that his name was misspelled on his tombstone.

What makes Teilhard a real hero in my book is not just that he told the truth and was eventually vindicated. What is so impressive is that he told the truth with love and with faith. Teilhard de Chardin never swerved in his loyalty to the Catholic Church or to the Society of Jesus. He was a hero of love and of faith.

We live in an age of the anti-hero. We seem to take great delight in exposing the tragic flaws in persons. It is good to keep in mind that there are still some incredibly heroic individuals in our midst.

DEATH

"Mighty Matt"

There has never been a child more eagerly awaited with joy than my nephew, Matthew Legere.

My brother Art and his wife Mary Jane wanted to conceive a child, and they were thrilled when they found out that they were pregnant. They broke the news to the rest of the family on Christmas day, and we all cried for joy.

During the nine months of the pregnancy, we directed to that baby about as much love as anyone could stand. We felt Mary Jane's tummy each week and were thrilled when we could feel the little one kicking away inside her.

Mary Jane must have set a record for baby showers. Everyone was so delighted to see her and Art so happy. All agreed that this young couple would be truly exceptional parents.

The delivery entailed complications. Mary Jane was in labor for three days. Art was present in the labor and delivery rooms all that time and the experience was extremely taxing to both of them. However, the anticipation of telephoning us with good news at the birth of the child made their ordeal a lot easier to bear.

The joyful phone call was never to be. When the doctors examined the newborn baby, they detected some problems. The full extent of the problems would come to light only gradually, but we knew within a day that the baby was born with some serious heart abnormalities.

If the child was a boy, they were going to name him either Matthew, which means "God's gift," or Christian. When the doctor told them that there were some difficulties, they looked at one another and said, "Well, I guess his name will be Matthew."

From the very beginning, Art and Mary Jane saw Matthew

not as a problem but as an opportunity. They knew that the whole family would grow as a result of God's gift. It was not easy for any of us. We all had to dig down inside ourselves and find out what we were made of. We found resources of strength and faith and love that we had never known we had.

The baby was a tough little guy. His parents nicknamed him "Mighty Matt." Throughout a series of surgical interventions, he fought for life with all his might. We like to think that he wanted to stay around so much because he had felt such intense love for him during those nine months in the womb.

During those first few weeks, we were all simply amazed by the faith perspective of his parents. Their attitude all along was, "He is not our child; he is God's child. If the Father wants to call him home, we will let him go. If he is meant to live, we will gladly take care of him."

Matthew lived a little more than a month before he went home to the Father. When Art and Mary Jane were told by the beautiful people at the Philadelphia Children's Hospital that their little bundle of love had died in the middle of the night, they accepted his passing as part of God's plan.

Consistent with their belief that Mighty Matt was not a problem but an opportunity, they gave his body to a team of scientists from U.C.L.A. There researchers were able to serve other children with heart defects as a result of what they found out by examining Matthew.

When we celebrated the Mass of the Angels for Matthew, it was a very special experience. We could actually feel the faith, hope, and love present in those assembled.

We could see that his life was a great success. So many persons were positively affected in so many ways. Though he lived only one month, Mighty Matt attained a goal that some fail to attain even in a long lifetime: He brought others together—in faith, hope, and love.

Not the Final Reality

"Ain't none of us gonna get out of it alive, Father." The school janitor told me that the other day, and it has been on my mind ever since.

So many of us run through life as if it were going to last forever. We are so bent on accomplishing things and impressing others that we lose sight of the fact that none of us is going to be around much more than seventy years.

Through elaborate makeup, plastic surgery, mod clothes, hair dye, vitamins, and exercise, we pursue the elusive goal of perpetual youth. We refuse to grow old gracefully. We seem determined to do everything in our power to squeeze every last day out of life.

When someone dies we all say, "What a shame!" It is almost as if we think that only the *unfortunate* die! We find it inconceivable to imagine ourselves one day lying there in the casket.

This unwillingness to come to terms with the reality of death is one of the things that makes us so nervous. Instead of seeing things in the context of eternity, we convince ourselves that the whole world will rise and fall on our ability in one short lifetime to accomplish this or that little project of ours. If we fail, we become tense and sometimes turn to drugs or alcohol or some other artificial outlet to help us cope with pressures and failures.

Christians are well-equipped to face the life-death question without becoming petrified. They know that death is the passageway to an eternal life with God. Death brings a certain natural sadness, but it should not be the sort of occurrence that causes us to come completely undone. Even the impending death of a loved one need not destroy us. Even our own death can be gracefully accepted. Obviously, the Christian will suffer like anyone else at the death of a loved one; it is just that our grief, as painful as it might be, is always seen in the context of the hope of Easter.

A few years ago I heard a priest friend of mine say that you do not really begin to live until you have accepted the fact of your own death. I believe this. Once you know you will die, and have accepted this fact on the gut level, then you are no longer afraid of anyone or anything. You can say what you believe and do what you are convinced is right, totally without fear of reprisal.

Furthermore, you will not worry yourself sick about what you are able or not able to accomplish in life. You know that you have only a few short years to live; you know that the Lord does not expect miracles of you; and you know that your salvation will be accomplished by your faith in Jesus Christ and not by how successful you were in this life.

The best example of a person who saw life in the proper perspective was Jesus Christ. Sometimes I ask myself, why did he wait until he was thirty years old before he began his public life? Why did he allow himself to be crucified after only three years of public ministry?

The answer to these questions is that Jesus accepted death as a *reality* but not the *final* reality. He knew that he would be with his Father for all eternity. So he was able to wait patiently for the acceptable time and then walk calmly into Jerusalem and say what had to be said, totally aware that his words would mean his death.

What mattered was not how long he lived, but what he did with his life.

Most of us need to fight constantly to keep things in context and remember that nothing on earth is worth getting an ulcer over. Life is short, and our daily problems are usually not all that significant.

So the next time I go to buy a jar of antacid, I hope I can keep in mind the words of our janitor, "Ain't none of us gonna get out of it alive."

Vanity of Vanities

Every so often I like to rummage around the attic of my family's home in Somerdale, New Jersey. The last time I did so I came across a box of my childhood memorabilia, gathering dust in the attic.

As a boy, I never thought that all my neat stuff would come to such an inglorious end. After all, my cub scout uniform, my collection of baseball cards, and my first altarboy cassock were pretty important to me at one time. Now, alas, these items have only sentimental value.

What material things are important to you? A collection of records, a fur coat, some jewelry, a college diploma, your father's watch, your mother's engagement ring?

Where will all our prized possessions be seventy-five years from now? Or, for that matter, where will we be seventy-five years from now? Unless we are very young, chances are we will all be dead and buried. The possessions that mean so much to us now will probably end up in a trash heap, or stored away in a dusty attic, or buried under a pile of junk in someone's basement.

Our prized possessions may then belong to someone who never knew us and cares not at all what we were like. As the author of the book of Ecclesiastes says, "All things are vanity!" (Ecclesiastes 1:2)

How many of us personally know others who had saved and hoarded every penny waiting for retirement, only to be disappointed when the big day came? They had let life pass them by; they had made no time for that sloppy love stuff. They had thought they were hardheaded realists. Then they discovered they had wasted their lives. Spending most of our energy acquiring material possessions—in youth, in middle age, or in old age—amounts to the same thing: vanity.

We may be as rich as Jean Paul Getty, but when we cash in our chips, it is all the same. We die and we cannot take it with us. I have yet to see a hearse followed by a U-Haul truck.

So we ask ourselves, "Does anything count in life?" Absolutely. Jesus tells us that life is full of value. The only trouble is that what Jesus and the church says is worthwhile, the world thinks is a waste of time. Kindness, generosity, fidelity, trust, commitment, patience, sensitivity, authenticity, cheerfulness, love—these are what makes life worth living. Those qualities and attitudes help to make a permanent change in our world.

Their impact cannot be so easily erased.

When a person throws a stone into a pool of water, ripples seem to go out from the point of impact forever. Once the spiritual values of kindness and love, fidelity and commitment enter our world, there is no stopping their effect.

As Christians we believe that we are on a winning team. The Spirit of Christ will continue to work among men and women. Eventually, his way of life will prevail.

The wise person knows this and lives accordingly. The foolish person, on the other hand, tries to support himself or herself with the material crutches that keep us going here on earth. One day we will have to stand before the Lord stripped of all those crutches. At that time we will not be able to fake it. Either we will be the high rollers who have accumulated a lot of worldly possessions, or we will be persons who have based their lives on values of the spirit.

A Beautiful Death

This is the story of the most beautiful death I have ever heard of. It is the story of the death of Father Jack Villano, a fifty-year-old pastor in the Camden diocese.

You may not think that fifty years is a very long life. But when a person has a history of heart troubles extending back to his early childhood, when that person had such a weak heart that no one ever thought he would make it to adulthood, when that person had his first heart attack at the age of twenty-nine, then fifty years is a long life. In point of fact, Jack considered it simply amazing that he made it that far. No one ever thought he would. But then Jack Villano had a way of frequently doing the unexpected.

The summer before his death marked a real milestone for him. He celebrated twenty-five years in the priesthood with a beautiful Mass for all his family and friends. Then he visited Europe for a few weeks. He loved every minute of it.

Almost immediately upon returning from Europe, he went

on a retreat with over twenty of his closest priest friends. Everyone loved the retreat, but Jack seemed to be especially moved. The retreat director, Sister Susanne Breckel, stressed the importance of human relationships. Sister Susanne is herself a victim of cancer, so her emphasis on the brevity of life and the importance of human love struck a responsive chord among the retreat participants.

One point that she made in particular really impressed Jack. She stressed the importance of telling those we love how much they mean to us. So moved was Jack that, when he returned from the retreat, he canceled all his appointments for the next week and spent the time visiting his closest friends to tell them, simply, that he loved them.

The following Sunday was the monthly meeting of our priest support group. We meet each month for an afternoon of prayer and sharing, followed by a meal together. This was one of Jack's favorite times of the month. He loved us all as brothers. Jack never missed a meeting. He was never happier than when he was with his friends in the priesthood.

After a couple of hours of deep sharing, Jack confided to the group that he had never been happier in his life. He said the retreat had put the missing piece in the jigsaw puzzle of his life. He said that for the first time he felt a complete sense of self-acceptance. He felt at peace with himself and with the world.

The room was getting warm. Jack walked down the stairs to turn on the air conditioner. He rejoined his brothers, sat down, gently put his head back—and died. The passing was so gentle, without the least indication of any discomfort whatever, that at first no one realized what had happened.

When we did realize that Jack had probably had a heart attack, one priest began to give him mouth-to-mouth resuscitation, another massaged his heart, and another called for an ambulance. But there was no pulse. Jack had gone home to the Father.

During his life Jack was seldom understood. That was because he was always ahead of his time. He was one of the first priests involved in liturgical renewal, the Cursillo movement, Charismatic Renewal, Marriage Encounter, and the like.

He was always in the vanguard of things. When I mentioned this to someone she said, "Then he must have suffered a lot." He did. Jack paid a high price for his prophetic insights.

Perhaps his incredibly beautiful death was the Father's way of saying, "Well done, good and faithful servant. Your gentle passing will be a sign to my people that individuals like you are close to my heart."

BODY/MIND/SPIRIT

The Body

"I could be more spiritual if only I could quit worrying about my body." If we have ever thought that way, it indicates that we have a misconception of the body's role as we grow in the Spirit.

The body is not an appendage, an obstacle to be overcome. The body is us. Every cell of our body is charged with Spirit. When we say that our body is a temple of the Holy Spirit, we do not mean that our body houses a vaporlike puff of smoke called a soul. The body is a dimension, the mind another, and the spirit still another. But the *person* is not fragmented that way. We *are* a body/soul/spirit. We are *one*.

Much of the misconception about the role of the body goes back to two heresies called Gnosticism and Manichaeism. The Gnostics and Manichaeans believed that the spirit was the noble part of the human body, whereas the body was corrupt and evil. These heresies contradicted the ancient Greek notion of the integration of body and spirit. The Greeks loved to sculpt the body and engage in sports and promote health of body, mind, and spirit; the Gnostics and Manichaeans advocated repressing anything having to do with the body, especially sex.

The "official" Judeo-Christian teaching on this matter has always been clear. The body is good. Bodily functions, including sex and reproduction, are good. In fact, everything God has created is good.

I put the word "official" in quotes because Gnostic and Manichaean tendencies have often crept back into the church's popular teaching about the body. One of the worst incursions in recent centuries was a heresy called Jansenism. Basically it was a warmed-over version of the old Manichaean hatred of the body. Jansenistic strains became fairly widespread in Europe, especially in France and Ireland. Because so many of the clergy that came to America were French or Irish, they brought with them this sick attitude toward the human body. Some clergy still have it.

Today, however, spirituality is recovering an appreciation for the role of the body. In particular, exercise, nutrition, and rest are seen as essential activities for the person who is serious about spiritual growth.

Exercise is very important. When we exercise vigorously, we bathe our cells with blood which has been nourished by fresh oxygen. We expel toxins through our breath and through our perspiration. We marvel at the miracle of movement and recapture the childlike quality of playfulness. A sluggish body, on the other hand, produces a sluggish mind and spirit. If you do not give your body its needed exercise, you do not properly love yourself, and your spirit will never be set free.

Nutrition in this country is a disaster. The additives and preservatives found in most foods contribute greatly to anxiety, hyperactivity, depression, cancer, and other disorders that are virtually unheard of among the American Indians and other spiritually sensitive cultures. In addition, we eat too fast, too much, and too thoughtlessly. We eat too much red meat and not enough fruit, grains, and vegetables.

Rest gives our body an opportunity to regenerate energy. If we drink coffee before we go to bed, or take unprescribed tranquilizers, or keep irregular hours, we are robbing our bodies of the deep rest needed so that we might renew ourselves properly.

Without a proper respect for the body, spiritual growth is virtually impossible.

Wholistic Medicine

A few years ago, a priest friend of mine from the Midwest asked his bishop if he could study medicine on a part-time basis. The bishop laughed him out of his office. But my friend was more on target than his bishop realized. There is a profound interrelationship among body, mind, and spirit.

As far back as 6000 B.C., there were physician-priests who treated all aspects of sickness. Gradually, due to specialization, the roles of physician and priest became separated. Within the last century further specialization has taken place with the emergence of psychiatrists to treat the mind.

Such specialization was inevitable, but humanity is slowly coming to the conviction that it is counterproductive to compartmentalize persons this way. Today we want to be treated as whole persons. This emphasis is called wholistic medicine. This new approach (which goes back to the ancients) is with us to stay.

Many doctors will tell you privately that sticking a needle in someone or prescribing some pills seldom gets to the source of the problem. It is merely treating symptoms. And because, according to estimates, up to eighty percent of all illnesses are psychosomatic, the doctor knows that he or she will be seeing the patient again shortly. A psychological or spiritual conflict, if left untreated, will undoubtedly manifest itself in some other symptom in a short time.

Wholistic medicine believes in treating people *before* they are sick. Wholistic doctors are more interested in facilitating health than in treating illness. The ancient Chinese had a similar approach. They would pay their doctor as long as they were healthy. As soon as they got sick, payment stopped. I wonder how such an idea would go over in this country!

The common objection to such a positive form of treatment is that doctors are too busy to spend time keeping persons healthy. They are already overworked treating sicknesses. Such a response, of course, begs the question. If we were healthier, there would not be so many of us lined up in the doctors' waiting rooms.

I suspect that at the heart of this whole dispute lies a basic unwillingness of many persons in the medical profession to share healing territory with anyone else. Once you admit that you do not have all the answers, then you lose your monopoly on the healing field.

Not long ago the cover of a national medical journal pictured doctors and nurses getting ready to perform an operation. Before beginning, they all had bowed their heads in prayer. Does that seem wrong or threatening to anyone? Well, in the next issue, the letters to the editor section was filled with violent outbursts from physicians who were furious at such a concession to witchcraft and mumbo jumbo. That is how nervous some doctors are when they see their healing monopoly being shared with anyone, even God.

But some other doctors are beginning to observe a crack in their cosmic egg. They are either dropping out of the American Medical Association entirely or at least maintaining a double affiliation with an honest-to-goodness alternative: the Academy of Holistic Medicine (AHM). This organization is composed of doctors, psychologists, ministers, and others in healing professions who want to treat the whole person.

The hardliners are still hanging in there. They debunk the laying on of hands, chiropractic, acupuncture, homeopathy, and wholistic healing, even though patients are discovering that they get results from these ancient and modern treatments, results that they do not get from a pill or a syringe.

It is not my intention to downplay doctors. I have the utmost respect for most of them. It is just that, in these exciting days in which we live, it is foolhardy for anyone to claim a monopoly on the truth.

Fasting and Wholeness

Fasting is a marvelous technique for influencing spiritual consciousness. Anyone seriously interested in pursuing the spiritual path should consider incorporating fasting into his or her spirituality.

Fasting is a practice found in all of the great religions of the world, including the Judeo-Christian tradition. Moses fasted for forty days before receiving the spiritual revelation that was the basis of the Ten Commandments. Jesus fasted for forty days before he began his public ministry. The prophet Mohammed goes so far as to say that fasting is the foundation of all religion.

Why, then, has fasting virtually disappeared from American Catholicism in recent years? In my opinion, the main reason is that the entire American church, including its leadership, has lost sight of the original goals, origins, and results of fasting.

Fasting was never designed to be a form of body hatred. It came into practice because spiritual devotees found that it heightened their consciousness, sharpened their mental faculties, and opened the psyche to spiritual experience. Fasting is not a punishment. It is an enjoyable experience. Besides cleansing the body of toxins, it helps us to think more clearly, and promotes positive emotions of faith, hope, and love.

What is the physiological explanation for all this? What is going on in the body when we are fasting? Apparently the parasympathetic autonomic nervous system (PANS) begins to dominate the functioning of the sympathetic nervous system (SANS). PANS controls positive emotions of peace and love; SANS seems to generate the negative emotions of doubt, guilt, anger, and hatred. We are usually dominated by SANS in our waking hours. PANS has more control when we sleep and when we fast.

Most persons are intimidated by fasting because they are accustomed to three meals each day. But the human body has an elaborate storage system built into its evolutionary structure. Our ancestors could not count on eating each day: poor hunting and occasional crop blight were facts of life. We simply do not need to eat every day.

How long can the human body go without eating (but not, of course, without liquids)? In the average person there are enough fat and toxins to burn for forty days before the body would begin to consume muscle tissues. Once I met a priest who had fasted for forty days (under a doctor's care) in the hope that his body would correct an infected gall bladder, thereby obviating the need for surgery. It worked.

It should be stated here very clearly that such a fast is

extreme and should never be undertaken without proper medical and spiritual supervision. In fact, *any* fast of a duration beyond twenty-four hours should be undertaken only with the utmost discretion and never without the proper consultation.

After that has been stated, however, it is likewise important to state that our bodies are bloated and poisoned with toxic substances. Moderate fasting that helps us get rid of these is good for the body and for the soul.

Some persons combine the spiritual benefits of fasting with other side benefits. Both Socrates and Plato fasted seven to ten days at a time to improve their mental abilities. There is a Bread for the World group in Camden, New Jersey, that fasts once a week so that it may sense a state of solidarity with the hungry of the world.

Why not consider returning to this ancient discipline? You will be doing it not to punish yourself but to try a technique that millions agree is an effective aid to spiritual growth.

Listening to the Body

One of the great things about the body is that it never lies. It is always trying to tell us something about ourselves.

Of course, sometimes the only message that the body has to communicate is that it has just caught the flu or some other communicable disease. With such illnesses, a person's mental condition has little to do with the discomfort that the body is experiencing.

Often, however, there is a very close connection between one's illness and the inner struggles one is going through. This is what is called a psychosomatic illness.

Sometimes persons mistakenly think that a psychosomatic illness is just a figment of one's mind. Nothing could be further from the truth. A psychosomatic illness is very real, but it is caused not by a virus, or wound, or infection, but by some inner turmoil that is bothering the person.

How common are these psychosomatic illnesses? I have

seen estimates that claim as much as eighty percent of our illness is of this nature. I heard one doctor say that he would have to close up shop if his work were confined solely to problems unrelated to the psyche.

The top five killers in this country are heart attacks, cancer, alcoholism, suicide, and accidents. Stress has been directly linked to heart attacks and indirectly linked to cancer. And it is pretty clear that alcoholism and suicide are associated with troubled personalities. Strangely enough, there is even a link between stress and accidents. Persons who are preoccupied are much more likely to be involved in serious accidents.

The message is clear: We should listen to our bodies. What are our bodies trying to tell us about what is going on inside us?

There is nothing morally wrong about having a psychosomatic illness. Its presence simply indicates that we do not have it "all together." It just means we are human.

I once did some research on the religious conversion of St. Augustine. Apparently he was a victim of a psychosomatic illness that affected his chest area. Augustine used to make his living with his lungs. He was a great teacher of rhetoric but gradually came to see his career as a hollow vocation.

As the moment of his conversion grew closer, the pain in his chest got more excruciating. It was almost as if his body were telling him that a life of rhetoric was not for him. Immediately after his conversion, his chest pain disappeared.

The two parts of my body that react to stress are my back and my stomach. When my work load gets too heavy, my back begins to tighten. This is my body telling me that what I am doing is "breaking my back." When I am facing an undesirable situation, my stomach begins to do flip-flops. This is my body telling me that I am having trouble "stomaching" the situation.

If we are serious about listening to our bodies, we should give them more time than just the few seconds we take before we pop a pill to assuage a symptom. I recommend dialoguing with the part of the body that is hurting.

An effective way to do this is by *writing*. Try speaking to the affected organ and ask what the problem is. Then put yourself in the role of the part that is hurting and write back to yourself. There is a hidden, subconscious wisdom in the body. The technique of writing is effective for some persons in helping to unlock this wisdom and bring it to consciousness.

It is common knowledge that we use only ten percent of our brain power. The more we learn to use the other ninety percent to our advantage, the better the chances are that we can gain some control over the psychosomatic illnesses that are destroying so many of us.

Beyond Body Language

Some years ago, the systematic study of body language was a real eye-opener to millions of persons. For the first time they could understand how human beings communicate nonverbally.

You may be familiar with some of the basic ideas. Folded arms, crossed legs, clenched fists often betray defensive attitudes. Arms at one's side or behind one's back may indicate an attitude of openness. The insight that we are *always* communicating with one another apparently rang true with the experience of most persons.

Today there is a new approach to understanding the human person that goes beyond body language. It is the theory that the shape and contours of our bodies have been caused by our emotional conditioning.

Our faces reveal what is going on inside us. For example, someone finds it a bit hard to believe that we are really happy when our face has a sour look. As John Powell, S.J., is always saying, "If you are happy, would you please inform your face?"

The theory under consideration, however, goes beyond just looking at the face and eyes of a person. It declares that the very shape of our body is making a visible statement about us. These ideas are outlined by Ken Dychtwald in his book *Body-*

Mind. The author says that there are five principal factors that influence the shape of our body.

The first factor is, of course, heredity. We inherit many bodily characteristics from our parents.

The second factor is physical activity. Even if they were dressed the same, we would normally not have any difficulty distinguishing a construction worker from a teacher. Working outdoors, pounding nails, lifting hundred-pound bags of cement—that kind of activity influences the shape of the body.

The third factor is nutrition. If we are heavy and puffy, for example, there is a good chance that we have sculpted our bodies this way by eating too much of the wrong foods.

The fourth factor is our environment. The streets of New Delhi, the wheat fields of Soviet Georgia and the island of Tahiti are three distinct environments that would influence the condition of our bodies in different ways.

The fifth factor is emotional and psychological activity and experience. By now, just about everyone recognizes that physical changes take place in our body as a result of our emotional state. For example, if I am nervous, I may feel "butterflies" in my stomach. If I am angry, my voice may rise, my heart may beat faster, and my muscles may stiffen.

The concept of body-mind accepts all this as a given and then goes on to suggest that any chronic emotional state may make permanent changes in the body.

For example, try re-creating in your body what happens when you are nervous or upset. How do the muscles in your stomach feel? Are you short of breath? Now ask yourself what would happen if you were nervous for a good part of each day. Surely, says Dychtwald, after months or years of exercising yourself in this way, the muscles in your belly and chest would begin to shape themselves to reflect this state of nervousness with its accompanying tensions and blockages.

Body-Mind shows how the shape of our spine, the thrust of our chin, the expansion of our chest, and the way we walk are all influenced by emotional and psychological factors.

Father Jack Villano, a deceased pastor in the Camden, New

Jersey, diocese, taught me while he was alive how to "own" all my feelings and emotions, and not blame them on anyone else. It looks as if the next step is to accept responsibility for even the shape and appearance of my own body.

Healing of Body and Spirit

Ever since the days of the Enlightenment there has been widespread mistrust between medicine and religion. Doctors have often judged the claims of religion to be unscientific, and church leaders have often been distrustful of science because it seemed that God was being left out of the picture.

But today there is dialogue between medicine and religion, in part because of important research in the area of psychosomatic illnesses. Doctors have always been aware that a good attitude toward life can color our emotions and brighten up a part of our day. But what about the stark reality of disease? Is our mental attitude partially responsible for the development of serious disease? And, even more interesting, can the powers of the mind contribute to the healing of diseases?

Kenneth R. Pelletier, Ph.D., assistant clinical professor at Langley Porter Neuropsychiatric Institute in San Francisco, is convinced that the human spirit does indeed profoundly influence our physical health. Dr. Pelletier wanted to know why a small percentage of individuals with "incurable" diseases somehow are healed of their illnesses. His personal interviews with a sampling of those who had been "miraculously cured" revealed the following findings.

All those who had recovered despite great odds had experienced:
- Profound intrapsychic changes. That is, their innermost being had been reshaped in some way by meditation, prayer, or some other spiritual practice.
- Profound interpersonal changes. Their relations with other persons had been placed on a new and more solid footing.
- Significant alterations in diet. These persons no longer took

their food for granted. They were conscious of nutrition and carefully watched what they ate.

● A deep sense of the spiritual, as opposed to the purely material, facets of life.

Dr. Pelletier is now convinced that a spiritual orientation in life actually improves one's physical health. He is by no means alone; countless other physicians have come to the same conclusion.

Psychologists, too, are coming to terms with the psychic benefits of true religion. In fact, there is a whole new school in psychology that is convinced a person cannot be a full human being without some openness to the religious dimension.

With medicine and psychology now comparing notes with religion, where do we go from here? It appears that the human endeavor may be on the brink of a great breakthrough. Instead of physicians and psychologists and clergy competing with one another, we may be in for a period of unprecedented cooperation. Religion will be seen as an equal partner in the healing professions.

Dr. David Breslan of the U.C.L.A. pain control unit notes that the ancient Chinese distinguished five levels of physicians: "Lowest was the veterinarian or animal doctor. Next came the doctor who used acupuncture to relieve specific complaints (symptomatic medicine). Third was the surgeon, who treated more serious health problems. Second highest was the nutritionist, who practiced preventive medicine by teaching what to eat. But highest of all was the philosopher-sage, who taught people the order of the universe. He was the only doctor who could directly effect a genuine cure, by going right to the heart of the problem: the patient's ignorance of how to live harmoniously with nature."

The Christian churches are in the unique position of being able to offer to the world the philosopher-sages whom it so desperately needs.

Thank God we are finally stopping our little Mickey Mouse wars with one another. A new age of cooperation is beginning among the healing professions. Religion will be playing a

crucial role in this endeavor. These are truly exciting times to
be alive!

SELF-INTEGRATION

Science and Religion Together

For a while the world's intelligentsia fondly hoped that human beings would eventually outgrow their addiction to religion. Science saw itself as the new, logical, realistic approach to reality. Religion was viewed as a collection of superstitions and fairy tales that catered to the ignorant masses. It was the goal of science eventually to liberate the human person from this pathetically unenlightened condition.

Many scientists have begun to have second thoughts about their judgment. They are reconsidering things for two reasons: a realization that science does not have all the answers, and a realization that true religion has humanizing—not dehumanizing—effects.

To say that science does not have all the answers is certainly an understatement. After determining that the human body is worth $1.25 and that love is merely the result of certain nerve stimuli, open-minded researchers know that they are far from understanding completely the human condition. There is a spiritual factor in the human person that science will never be able to measure. And apart from this inability to measure the spiritual dimension of the human person, there is the added factor of the harm that is caused when research is carried out in a context devoid of human values.

The same technology that has brought the blessings of electricity and immunity from diseases has also brought us the curses of the atomic bomb, germ warfare, napalm, acid rain, and such morally complex possibilities as sex-change operations.

Without spiritual values to guide us, the human race may, without any exaggeration, literally self-destruct by the turn of the century.

Even hard-nosed, logical scientists are aware that they have made some incredibly tragic mistakes. They are now crying out for ethical principles with which to carry on their research. The other basis of collaboration between science and religion is the realization that true religion makes for healthier human beings.

The "humanist" school of psychology decided to study healthy persons, to see what makes them tick. Freud, by contrast, concentrated on pathological individuals in his society, to see what made them miss a tick here and there.

Erich Fromm, Rollo May, Paul Tillich, and other humanists found that most of the healthy individuals they studied believed in God and had a system of moral values. For years scientists had been working under the assumption that religion was only for neurotics. And here the humanists concluded that the real neurotics were the ones who were devoid of religious faith!

Scientists have really come unglued with the increasing evidence that mental telepathy, telekinesis, ESP, levitation, healings, visions and other psychic phenomena really do take place. And the icing on the cake was provided when studies found that prayer and meditation actually have physically beneficial side effects.

The world needs scientific research. The world also needs encounter with God and the humanizing values that flow from such an encounter.

Jung at Heart

Anyone with even the slightest interest in the relationship between religion and the human mind should be acquainted with the work of Swiss psychologist Carl Jung. Jung was originally a disciple of Sigmund Freud, but he went his separate way over the issue of the role of religion in mental health.

Freud was convinced religion was damaging to mental health. It fostered reliance on some father figure somewhere up in the clouds. Religion made the human person less fully human and less mature. It was a factor contributing to mental illness.

Jung could not have disagreed more with his mentor. Jung concluded that religious symbols were innate in persons' minds. When we are born, our mind is not a blank slate but already contains the seeds of religious symbolism. Jung called these powerful religious symbols with which we are born "archetypes." It was his conclusion after fifty years of clinical practice that no one could escape the need to come to terms with these archetypes.

For example, he found that all persons are born with a God archetype in their minds. To achieve mental health they must come to terms with God in their lives.

Whether this God archetype actually exists apart from the human mind is a separate question. Jung said that as a Christian he believed that God is a reality. But as a clinical psychologist he was absolutely certain that persons had to live *as if* God exists.

Such basic patterns of the human mind must be taken seriously. Jung concluded that if persons tried to deny the existence of God in their own lives, they were heading toward neurosis and even in some cases total psychosis.

Jung observed a whole generation of persons who were trying to live their lives as if they were free to reject arbitrarily these basic patterns of the human mind. He observed that, of all the persons he had dealt with from all over the world, he never came across one person over thirty-five years of age whose mental problem was not fundamentally "religious" in nature.

A more recent example of what Jung was trying to get across can be found in the film *Close Encounters of the Third Kind*. The main character has in his mind an image of a mountain that he simply must come to terms with. He is not sure how it got there or what it means. He just knows he must pursue it if he is ever to have peace of mind. His family thinks he is crazy, but that does not deter him. Certain quests in life must be pursued no matter what anyone else thinks and even if one has to go it alone.

According to Jung, the image of God that we all have in our minds is like that mountain. We are not sure how it got there, and sometimes we are not sure what it means. We are just somehow aware that we will not possess inner peace until we pursue our quest for God.

The quest is a lonely one, to be sure. We must go it alone, and many will misunderstand what we are about. But the quest for the living God is for us simply irresistible.

We can thank Carl Jung for putting the religious quest into terminology the twentieth century can understand. But at a deeper level, we must thank our God who is the very source of that quest.

God and Ego

The ego has been getting a lot of bad press lately. Some speak as if the ego were some sort of deterrent to spiritual growth. Actually, the development of a strong ego is an absolute prerequisite for mental and spiritual health.

The ego is what gives us a foothold in life. We begin life's journey not even knowing the difference between ourself and our mother. We do not know who we are. The ego helps us establish an identity.

If you want to experience just how tenuous our foothold in life really is, try telling a little boy that he has a different name from the one he actually has. The boy will probably begin to panic. The child panics because he is not really convinced that he knows who he is.

The first twenty-five years or so of a life are dedicated to helping an individual establish this tenuous foothold in life. Many are never able to complete the process. In extreme cases, they end up being hospitalized for psychosis. Psychosis involves a split with reality. The psychotic is lost in his or her own inner world, which often makes complete sense to him or her (but not to anyone else).

In less extreme but far more common cases, the individual is able to function in society by completely identifying with group thinking. The person's identity is totally dependent on family, local community, church, and nation. Such a person is, as T. S. Eliot said, one of the "hollow men" of society. They are like zombies, the walking dead. They are locked into a state of immature dependency on group thinking.

Many of our greatest saints were men and women with strong and healthy egos. Augustine, Ignatius of Loyola, Teresa of Avila, and Catherine of Siena are only a few of our better known saints who had a strong sense of their identity and their spiritual gifts. Thomas Merton, Dorothy Day, and Mother Teresa are contemporary examples of the same kind of person.

But wait a minute. During a spiritual journey, is not the ego supposed to die? Not exactly. What is supposed to happen is that the ego, once it has well established itself in reality, is called to put itself at the service of one's higher self. To do this, the ego has to undergo a kind of death, to surrender control to this higher power. It is not exactly a death, but it surely feels like it!

St. Paul gives us a good example of such a transformed personality when he says, "I live, no longer I, but Christ lives in me." Notice that the ego has not been eliminated entirely. He still distinguishes between "Christ" and "I." If he had killed his ego, he would say, "No, my name is not Paul. My name is Jesus Christ."

What we are aiming for, then, is not the destruction of the ego but its transformation. Carl Jung felt very strongly about our need to maintain a healthy sense of ego. That is one of the reasons he considered it unwise for Westerners to immerse themselves in Eastern religions.

The spiritual ideal of the East is to lose oneself in the All, as a drop of water in the ocean. In the West, on the other hand, the highest state of spiritual union has been portrayed as a "mystical marriage" between the soul and God.

I come into contact with a lot of persons who want to hurry into a deep union with God. Of course, that is our *ultimate* goal. But an absolutely necessary step in this journey is the development of a strong and healthy ego. Those who try to bypass this step, will inevitably end up as robots. The glory of God is not a zombie, but a person fully alive.

God and Superego

One of the main reasons why many persons are afraid to pray is that prayer in the past has left them with bad feelings. This frequently happens when individuals confuse God with their own superego.

If Jesus taught us anything, it is that we are all loved unconditionally by the Father. This is point one. No matter what sin we have committed or are contemplating, the Father always smiles on us. The sin harms us, it does not harm God. Our God, as St. John tells us, is love.

The superego, on the other hand, is not so understanding. The superego is the "voice" within us that screams oughts and shoulds at us. The superego plays all of the old "bad boy" and "naughty girl" tapes that we picked up during childhood. Gestalt therapy calls it our "super top dog." Transactional Analysis calls it our "critical parent." Religion has often mistakenly called it our "conscience."

The superego has a temporary role to play in our development as persons. After all, we cannot expect children to make adult decisions. We have to give children an unambiguous set of guidelines for their own protection.

We never erase the tapes we were given by our superego. What we have to do is to acquire a different set of tapes that speak the message of Jesus and to play these new tapes at a louder volume than the old superego tapes.

The new set of tapes is not just based on wishful thinking. Good theology tells us that we are made in the image and likeness of God. With the passage of time, and with God's grace, we can come to discover what is called "Christ consciousness." This amounts to the amazing discovery that we are actually called to live the life of the Trinity. By finding Christ within, we are led to the Father by the power of the Spirit.

This inner journey can be a rough one; we may have to cross a few minefields before we can discover springs of living water. Before we can dig out our treasure within, we may have to dispose of a lot of garbage beneath the surface of our consciousness.

One thing that scares persons off from the spiritual journey is this onslaught of repressed ugliness that confronts us when we begin to look within. All kinds of forces and voices smack us in the face. One of the first voices to do so is that old superego that has been hanging around since childhood.

At that point, persons frequently make a critical mistake. They identify God with their superego and make a quick decision to scurry back to the surface of life. Who can blame them? After all, if God is nothing but a critical parent laying a load of guilt, oughts, and shoulds on us, who in his or her right mind needs God?

How can you tell which is God and which is the superego? When the voice of God is speaking to us, we do not feel trapped and backed into a corner. We are gently invited to grow, not browbeaten and made to feel unworthy. The feeling is one of being shown possibilities rather than being issued an ultimatum.

Our old nemesis the superego, on the other hand, is a relentless taskmaster. We feel like we have no choice open to us. We *must, ought, should* do such and such. There is no inner peace and no feeling of freedom.

What a pity so many persons think that by rejecting their superego they are rejecting God! In rejecting their superego, they may be closer to the kingdom of heaven than they suspect.

Multiple Selves

Back in 1976, while I was in the midst of a spiritual crisis, someone gave me an insight that I have never forgotten. Professor Ewert Cousins of Fordham University told me that we all have a true self and a false self.

This made no sense to me at the time. It seemed he was advocating some sort of spiritual schizophrenia. But over the last several years I have come to see that we have many subpersonalities.

There are many psychological systems that try to sort out the various images we have of ourselves. My favorite system is that of Dr. Karen Horney. She speaks of our having four selves: the real self, the actual self, the despised self, and the idealized self.

The *real* self is who we are potentially, if we are not neurotic. This is the way God sees us. As far as God is concerned, we are all created good and in his image and likeness. This is our Christ-self, our true self, our God-self. This is the self that is healthy and whole and free.

The *actual* self is who we are actually, with our individualized package of health and unhealth. Jesus was the only one who was all he was potentially able to be; the rest of us fall into the category of being somewhat free and somewhat neurotic. We are all *in process*; we are all *becoming*; we are all *not yet.*

The *despised* self is the neurotic voice of self-condemnation. This is the bully within us, the cruel taskmaster that is never satisfied no matter what we do. This is the voice of the shoulds and oughts and shalt-nots. The despised self loves to accuse and condemn and "put down."

Finally, the *idealized* self is the way we have always dreamed we could be. This is the self that leads us to delusions of grandeur. Sometimes there is a great discrepancy between how we actually are and how we see ourselves in our Mitty-esque flights of fancy.

First to go should be the *idealized* self. It is absolutely self-defeating to pursue pipe dreams that have no relation to reality. Unrealistic expectations that we impose upon ourselves are often based on nothing but blatant pride.

Debunking the *despised* self is a little tougher. Like the idealized self, it tries to tell us that putting down the actual self is based on noble motives and deep humility. Actually, it is our old nemesis pride again. It wants us to believe more in our personal unworthiness than in the God who has redeemed us.

What about the *real* self? We will have no problem as long as we understand that the real self is a result of God's grace. We will have difficulty, though, if we do not have a true picture of the real self and we begin to pursue an impossible image of ourselves. We will almost certainly be off on another self-hatred excursion when we do not measure up. We all have the life of Christ inside us, but we are courting disaster if we try to make believe that we are Jesus Christ incarnate.

Mental and spiritual health come only when we accept our actual selves as we are, with all of our blemishes and sinful tendencies. We accept ourselves simply because we believe more in the power of the risen Christ than we do in our own weakness.

PROBLEMS

Seeking Religious Experience

It is not much fun being lonely. Consequently, human beings have devised various techniques and systems to help them feel a part of something larger than themselves. When persons do in fact experience a profound union with nature or with that ultimate reality we call God, they have had what is loosely termed a religious experience.

Everyone seeks religious experience. What we often settle for, however, is considerably less than the ultimate.

One of the most common ways persons feel a sense of belonging is by identification with a nation. If you were asked to write down five things that you are, chances are one of those things you would write down would be "an American."

Our national pride was hurt by the hostage situation in Iran. Americans felt that to demean one soldier or one state official is to attack the whole populace. This form of group consciousness enables some individuals to attain some slight liberation from the tyranny of the ego.

Another attempt at escaping from loneliness is identification with a sports team. Identity with their local teams is so great that fans are elated when they win and take it personally when they lose. If their team does not make it to the World Series, the whole city will go into mourning.

Sexual love and jogging are two more ways that some have of overcoming loneliness. Sexual union is the most common way for persons to escape the narrow confines of their egos. Jogging too is becoming an increasingly popular source of ego transcendence. Long-distance runners eventually move beyond an obsession with their stopwatches and beyond using jogging merely as a means to improve their appearance or stretch their lifespan.

When someone recently remarked to me that my running would add ten years to my life, I was unable to relate to that observation. I run for quality of life, not quantity. Specifically, I run because I frequently experience a real sense of union with nature and with God. That is no small thing. However, realizing that reformed drinkers, recently born-again Christians, and turned-on joggers are more likely to turn people off than to convert anyone, let me quickly move on.

Two potentially harmful tactics of ego transcendence are alcohol and other drugs. Some drink and take other drugs because it momentarily expands their consciousness. Alcohol allows deeper truths about oneself to come to the surface. Shy persons become bullies and bullies become lovers. Drinkers often feel good about themselves. But alcohol is dangerous, of course, because it can and does addict millions of persons. It also kills. Cirrhosis of the liver is one of the five major killers in our country. About half of all fatal automobile accidents involve drinking.

It is the same with other drugs. They may give their users a momentary release from anxiety, or chemically induced courage, or even mystical insight. But drugs are dangerous because they too can be physically or psychologically addictive. Also, they pollute the human body and may lead to all sorts of destructive behavior.

Which brings us back to the best and most natural form of ego transcendence: religion. Not the weekend crash courses in mystical enlightenment, but the time-tested and proven religions of the world. For us, Christianity, specifically Catholicism, is psychologically sound and is designed and equipped to lead a person to love of oneself, others, the cosmos, and God.

There is nothing wrong with being an American or a sports fan. The natural ecstasies are there to be enjoyed, too. But nothing will help us overcome a sense of loneliness like really getting into the wealth of our religious tradition.

Stealing Fire

It is easy to understand someone who rebels against God

directly. After all, our egos all desire to be gods unto themselves. When some persons say that they would rather rule in hell than serve in heaven, we know exactly what they are talking about.

But there is another, less direct way of rebelling against God. It is much more subtle, and "religious" persons are the ones who use it most frequently. I call it "stealing fire" from God.

Prometheus was a famous figure in Greek mythology. He got into trouble because he tried to sneak up on the gods and steal some of their fire. He was not foolish enough to utter a direct challenge to the gods. He just wanted to get a little of what they had and use it for his own egocentric purposes.

This sort of mentality is deadly for the Christian, for it tries to reduce God to the status of a miserly old grinch who does not want to share what he has. When we "win" our salvation, it is we who think we have outfoxed God. In playing this little game, we try to reduce God to our own level.

Authentic spiritual insight tells us that there is, in fact, nothing to "win" at all. There is only God. We, apart from God, do not even exist. No real opposition to God is possible, in the long run, because there is no independently existing "we" to do any opposing.

Promethean man or woman is afraid of the giftedness of life. If God's life is a true gift, then there is nothing to gain or win. There is no battle and no independent cast of characters. There is only God.

Because the ego wants to be something in itself, it keeps looking for a fight—anything at all to give it the illusion of independent existence.

One of the more common ways of "stealing fire" is by allowing ourselves to give in to guilt. The false self loves guilt because it assumes that there is an independent "I" that is feeling guilty about offending another independent being: God.

Guilt is a trick of the false self. It is a way of avoiding the kingdom of heaven within us. As Thomas Merton puts it,

"Perhaps I am most afraid of the strength of God in me. Perhaps I would rather be guilty and weak in myself than strong in him whom I cannot understand."

Guilt reinforces the idea of separation. The guilty person is content in a strange sort of way because at least his or her autonomy is safeguarded. That is what the ego craves: separation and autonomy.

Conversion has to do with seeing oneself in a larger field of reference, the only field of reference that ultimately exists. Conversion implies turning away from guilt. This is not repression, and it certainly does not imply having it all together. It has to do simply with letting go and "letting God be God."

The great moment comes when we finally stop trying to experience God as doing something beneficial for us. It comes when we quit trying to gain heaven and quit even trying to be holy. We wake up when we realize that there is only God, and God is love. We will be happy and real only when we become extensions of God's love.

This trick the ego plays is at the same time complicated and simple. I know that I have been fooled at times into trying to "steal fire" from the gods. Have you?

False Psychics

If anything is mortally sinful, it is using spiritual gifts for personal profit. Yet this sort of religious rip-off is taking place with increasing frequency these days. I am referring specifically to the psychic charlatans who are making a handsome profit by duping the spiritually gullible.

If you plunk down the required fee, you can have your aura or your palm read, get a life reading, or hear your fortune told by Egyptian tarot cards. Gullible clients forget to read the small print, the words of disclaimer that usually accompany these shams: "The show is for entertainment purposes only."

To be sure, I believe that many individuals do have psychic gifts. Examples of clairvoyance, mental telepathy, healing, dream interpretation, and extrasensory perception abound in the Scriptures. They abound today, too. It is just that we badly need some discernment in this area.

One extreme is to deny outright the validity of such phenomena or to attribute them to the work of Satan. This is the attitude of the fundamentalist. The other extreme is to follow every self-styled guru who comes along. This is the attitude of the fool. We need an open mind in this area, but an open mind is not the same thing as a hole in the head. It is crucial that we "try the spirits to see whether they be of God" (1 John 4:1).

What criteria can we use to judge all these psychic phenomena? First, it is safe to discount any so-called psychics appearing on talk shows, or in the central corridors of shopping malls, or in local watering holes. Psychics genuinely gifted by God do not allow their gifts to be commercially exploited in such a cheap and tawdry manner.

Second, look at the humility level of the person. Any true psychic is aware that the power is coming from a source beyond his or her puny ego. So if the person has a big head, forget it. But if the person in question sincerely gives the credit to God, then you can move on to the third and most important test.

Most critical is the psychic's love level. Does the person radiate love? Is the gift being used for the service of others? Does the psychic have a genuine love for himself or herself, others, the cosmos, and God? If the answer to these questions is yes, you may be in the presence of an individual who has been gifted by God for the good of his people. We should respect such a person.

Recently I had the privilege of meeting a group of genuine Christian psychics. They have come to accept as normal what most of us consider to be abnormal or positively weird. But the great thing about these persons was that they were so humble and full of love. No power seeking. No commercial exploitation. But plenty of love. I have never met a friendlier, more accepting, more wholesome group of persons in my life.

There is plenty of room in our churches for such spiritually gifted persons. In fact there is even a Catholic-oriented study group called Imago Mundi that concerns itself with paranormal experiences. What a shame it is when gifted individuals encounter opposition from narrow-minded critics who simply do not understand that God is free to operate in our lives in whatever way he chooses.

Once again, discernment is always necessary. If some character wants to sell you a "long-distance psychic message" for $25, be suspicious. But if you encounter a humble, loving person with genuine psychic gifts, count yourself privileged.

Negativism

Nothing destroys a community more effectively than does a spirit of negativism. When we become possessed by this destructive tendency, we can destroy relationships and individuals with devastating swiftness and effectiveness.

It is always much easier to tear down than it is to build up. When we love, we build slowly—one brick at a time. But when we unleash the powers of negativism, we demolish an edifice with one fell swoop.

Just try saying something positive in a group. How many others pick up on it? But start playing the "ain't it awful" game, and everyone wants to play. Hours can pass by while we lament all the mistakes that "they" are making. We lick our chops as we assassinate characters and criticize all individual efforts by anyone creative or visionary.

Psychologists tell us we act this way because we have not yet integrated our own "shadow." All of us have unsavory aspects of our personalities that we are not proud of. Rather than face and accept the antisocial and primitive parts of ourselves, we "project" them onto others. Laying all the blame for the world's problems on "them" enables us momentarily to avoid coming to terms with who we are.

A Pollyanna approach to reality, on the other hand, is just as undesirable. Persons who walk around with a plastic smile always glued on their faces are just as much out of touch. It is a rough world we live in; there are many crazy things happening out there. It is not unchristian to take note of and discuss such things. It becomes unchristian and dehumanizing only when we lose our center and become swept up in negativism.

Any statement we make to others should be made with love and compassion. It can still be constructively critical, of course, but it should be made dispassionately and with sensitivity.

Why is it so important to work toward wholeness and against rampant negativism? Quite simply because a spirit of negativism destroys all who come into contact with it. The community or relationship being torn apart obviously suffers. But frequently overlooked is the fact that negativism also eventually destroys the one who thinks and speaks negatively.

Doctors estimate that the great majority of their cases are psychosomatic in nature. Remember that a psychosomatic illness is not something imaginary. It is very, very real. It is just that it has been caused by emotional or spiritual disharmony. The body eventually shows the effects of negative factors that have been consuming a person's psyche.

Not all criticism is destructive. Some of it is positively beneficial. The most valuable critic of our society or our church is a prayerful person. Truly prayerful persons are humble and compassionate. They are humble because they have made their own inner journey and have faced up to the enemy within. They are compassionate because they now recognize how weak and inconsistent we all are. Honed away are the rough edges of self-righteousness. Always implicit in any constructively critical comment is a sense of "there but for the grace of God go I." There is much less projection and much more true insight.

I am all for responsibly evaluating the situation in which we find ourselves. But a lot of our negative judgments come from unresolved areas of our own psyches. It is only after we have faced ourselves honestly that we are qualified to make any meaningful judgments about our world. Self-pitiers deserve only our pity. Prayerful persons are the only ones who can speak with any credibility about what is wrong with our world.

The Shadow Knows

One of the reasons for the popularity of *Star Wars, E.T.*, and other space-age westerns is that America is starved for heroes. The movies happily provide us with the noble, altruistic, good guys we so desperately need.

But such all-perfect heroes exist only on the screen or in our imaginations. And it is not much fun to come to this realization. In fact the last twenty years or so have been rather painful ones for Americans. We have found out that our society is racist, our armies are vincible, and our politicians are capable of atrocious crimes against the populace. We have caught the CIA testing nerve gas on U.S. citizens, the FBI illegally listening to our phone conversations, a president trying in vain to convince us he was not a malefactor, and persons in the Pentagon planning seriously for nuclear war.

All these revelations have been disillusioning. Our age of innocence has come to an end. We now know that even national heroes have their Achilles' heel. If investigators are inclined to look for a chink in the human armor, they will eventually find it.

But, to tell the truth, yanking our heroes down from their pedestals has also been a lot of fun for many of us. For when we self-righteously point the finger at others, we can, at least momentarily, avoid taking a good, hard look at our own tendencies to evil.

The important word here is momentarily. Because eventually our "shadow" knocks on the door of our heart and demands to be recognized. If we steadfastly deny its existence and insist on denying the destructive part of our psyche, the tension of living such a lie will eventually drive us to drink, or drugs, or some other form of neurotic or psychotic behavior.

Healthy persons are humbly aware that they are made of flesh and blood, are amazingly weak, and are capable, but for

God's grace, of almost any evil.

But who wants to admit that? We would much rather identify ourselves with the good guys. That is because we all have an "idealized self" that we wish to project. As a goal, that is fine. And if others put us on a pedestal, there is not much we can do about it. The fatal mistake is in believing that we really are that "idealized self." For when we begin to lose touch with ourselves and begin proudly inhaling others' compliments, we are setting ourselves up for a colossal crash.

The best way to avoid all this is to take an honest look at ourselves with the complete confidence that Christ can redeem every part of us. The Lord never dealt harshly with greed, sins of the flesh, sloth, or other capital sins. When we can admit to ourselves these repressed areas and tendencies, the Lord with his healing love can restore us to a sense of wholeness.

The only deadly sin is the sin against the Holy Spirit: pride. That sin is deadly because we try to talk ourselves out of the need for redemption. We refuse to acknowledge our own creaturehood and place ourselves on the level of God himself. "There is nothing wrong with me; it is the others who need healing."

Carl Jung was convinced that meeting our own shadow is necessary not just for our own mental health but for the future existence of humanity. The Germans, for example, were unable to face their collective shadow, and they projected their guilt onto the Jews. The whites in America have done a similar thing by projecting their own primal instincts onto blacks.

It is only when we can integrate ourselves into Christ that we will reach a sense of wholeness. For Jesus died on a cross that was anchored in the earth and pointed to heaven. He was flanked by a bad thief and a good one. He is certainly capable of helping us to accept our whole selves. Even our shadow.

The Devil in Us

Poltergeist. Swamp Thing. Demon possessed children and

chainsaw massacres. Killer birds, sharks, and whales. What is possessing our national consciousness? Have we gone completely crazy?

Not really. All this fascination with the occult and with hideous violence is the most natural thing for our society. It is natural and inevitable inasmuch as we as a society are almost completely incapable of handling our own inner monsters.

Let me explain. Persons have always known that there are destructive forces at work in their psyches. This was the viewpoint of Jesus, the early church, and almost anyone who has really been in touch with what is going on in his or her mind.

Jesus spoke often of an autonomous, independent agency opposed to love. He called this agency "Satan," making it clear that the force was real and personal and not just the impersonal absence of good.

If you think Jesus was merely speaking out of a limited worldview, think again. Most depth psychologists believe that Jesus' understanding of the spiritual world was profound. He knew what he was talking about when he warned us of the dangers of the Evil One.

Of course—and this is very important—most of what we think is devilish *inside us* is only the result of our inner fragmentation. Some fundamentalists attribute *every* sin to a willful collusion with Satan. Many of them eventually break down. Such a burden of being totally responsible for our own incompleteness is simply too much for them to carry.

According to priest-psychologist John Sanford, we must distinguish between chaotic or undifferentiated fragments of our personality, which may seem to us to be devilish but which must be included in our personalities, and absolute or ultimate evil. The latter is to be feared. But the former—our bad habits and personality problems and sins of weakness—are to be handled with patience, compassion, and a good sense of humor. We need to make peace with our weak human nature. Our weaknesses may, in God's providence, even help to round out our personalities.

But the common wisdom of our age does not even get this

far. Millions of persons are so out of touch with themselves that they even deny their personalities are fragmented. "Everything is fine, thank you. I'm okay. I'm one of the good guys with the white hats. There are no negative forces within me. That's all in the imagination. I'm in total control of what I think and do. Bad dreams are the result of eating before going to bed. Criminals are genetically inferior. Everything I do and think is done with the highest and purest motivation."

Our deepest selves instinctively rebel at such nonsense. Our negative forces demand to be dealt with. But because we lack the courage to look within, we subconsciously "project" all our fears of the unknown onto celluloid images that help us handle the inner demons we are incapable of facing. We compensate for our inability to deal with the threatening unknown by screaming and squirming at the poor demons and beings that cavort across our movie and television screens.

This would be great if we were little kids. It is healthy for youngsters to be fascinated with stories like Little Red Riding Hood and the big, bad wolf. Such stories give children something concrete to focus on. It helps them deal with their fears of the known and the unknown.

But we are supposed to be grown up. We are *not,* of course, and that is the point. We are still spiritual, mental, and emotional midgets.

Have we seen the last of the horror movies? Not by a long shot. They will continue to proliferate until we get the courage to take a good, honest, compassionate look within ourselves, and deal with what is really there.

Burnout

If you are feeling depleted, out of energy, and unable to reanimate yourself, you may be a victim of "burnout."

Burnout can happen to persons in any walk of life, but it is most common among those in the helping and healing professions. It is closely related to stress and may last for years.

First-degree burnout is the mildest stage. It is characterized by frequent short-lived bouts of irritability, fatigue, worry, and frustration. It affects our performance, but we usually can at least cope with things.

Second-degree burnout has the same basic symptoms as the above, but the difference is that now the symptoms last for two weeks or more. Anyone can have a bad day, or two or three bad days, or even a bad week. That is to be expected at times. But when we start having a number of bad weeks, a bad month, or a bad year . . . chances are we have a serious problem on our hands.

Third-degree burnout is yet more serious. The body begins to act out the psychic or spiritual problem we are experiencing. One of the great things about the body is that it never lies. Thus, when psychosomatic illnesses begin to appear, we are usually *forced* to admit that something is seriously wrong.

Among the illnesses that are often psychosomatic are ulcers, gastrointestinal problems, chronic back pain, migraine headaches, colitis, asthma, sexual impotence, loss of appetite, and high blood pressure. Such illnesses may be a blessing in disguise, *if* they finally prompt us to do something about our lifestyle.

Specifically, how do persons feel when they are at the initial stages of "burnout"? Physically, the feeling is one of being worn out, listless, and subject to frequent colds and viruses. Psychologically the "burnout" victim experiences an increased distancing from work, and has an abiding suspicion that "everyone wants to get a piece of me, and there is not enough of me to go around." Spiritually, the "burnout" victim begins to lose hope and begins to question his or her own goodness and the goodness of those he or she lives or works with.

How do we deal with "burnout" when it strikes? Volumes are being written on this, but here let us just take a quick look at a couple of preliminary steps that would be wise.

First of all, learn to recognize the symptoms when they occur. Do some reading. Familiarize yourself with the various symptoms, so that if they occur, you will not think you are cracking up.

Secondly, face the symptoms and accept personal responsibility for getting better. Do not rely on diversionary tactics such as overeating, excessive drinking, taking tranquilizers, or withdrawing from family and friends.

Finally, realize that you are responsible only for how you respond to the various stresses in your life. Many external factors are beyond your control. In other words, you are not the Messiah. If you try to take the responsibilities of the world on your shoulders, you will inevitably be crushed.

Practical steps will flow from an attitude of trust and existential humility. The "burnout" victim simply has to learn how to slow down and relax.

The psychosomatically ill, as well as the millions of mentally crippled persons in our country, are part of the fallout from the crazy, stress-filled society in which we live. We are not able to change the world to make it suit our fancy. But we can learn to take responsibility for the way we react to our world.

PRACTICES

Spiritual Journal

If you are capable of being reasonably honest with yourself, and if you believe in God's unconditional love for you, please read on. Otherwise, try something else besides keeping a spiritual journal.

You do not have to be a saint to use this technique for spiritual growth. You have only to believe that you could be the object of personal love.

Several years ago a priest friend tried to introduce me to this technique. I had learned a similar technique in another context, and I liked to write anyhow. But I wanted no part in writing a simple letter to the Lord each day. I did not like the technique because I was afraid of the honesty it required. But now that I have come to experience the unconditional love of the Father, I look forward each day to this practice.

Anyone can use this technique. It is not necessary to consult a confessor or spiritual director or anyone else beforehand. If you can write a letter, you can give it a try.

Of course, writing such a letter for the first time may give you a very strange sensation. You are not sure if you are talking to God or talking to yourself. Once you get into it, though, it is not so strange as it might sound.

Courses on this technique are available in some parishes, and they can give you an in-depth approach to the subject. Here I want only to share a few of my own experiences with this spiritual exercise.

I write in my journal first thing in the morning and right before I go to bed. In the morning I simply jot down as much of my dreams as I can remember. At night I review the day in writing. My aim is to write without listening to my inner censor that rationalizes and explains things away before I even face them. Instead, I ask myself "How did I feel when this was happening? What do I think God was trying to tell me today?" Honesty is the key.

What are the benefits of this strange practice? Obviously, different persons are likely to derive different benefits from daily use of the spiritual journal. But two things that most persons seem to find are direction and perspective.

We tend to get sucked into the maelstrom of activities that encircles us, and we are not sure we are going anywhere. Often we are content to just scrape through one more day. But with journal writing I can often see a definite direction unfolding in my life. I flip back to my entry of several months ago and I see there the seeds of my present frame of mind. I discern a common thread showing me that Someone is directing the course of my life. To know experientially that I am not in this game of life alone is no small thing indeed.

Perspective is another benefit I derive from journal writing. Some days it seems as if the whole world is crashing in on me. I am not sure I can cope, and I am convinced that I will never be able to get out of the quicksand in which I find myself. I write it down in my journal, half expecting an earthquake to cap a perfectly horrendous day. But when I look back at that entry on a sunny day later on, I smile to myself and am forced to conclude that many of my disastrous situations are cured, after all, by a good night's sleep.

Keeping a spiritual journal will not solve all our problems. But many of us find that it helps us as we walk down the hazardous road of life. Try it; it may help you.

What Good Are Dreams?

When was the last time you heard a sermon on dreams? Probably never.

There is nothing about dreams in the Baltimore Catechism or the documents of Vatican II. But dreams play an extremely important role in both the Old and New Testaments. And they also play an extremely important role in contemporary psychotherapy. So why have they been ignored by the church?

Probably the answer is that we have goofed. We have tried to be up-to-date and have fallen into the trap of believing that the only valid knowledge is scientific knowledge. We are afraid of dreams. We ignore their spiritual import because the predominant spirit of the age ignores them.

How foolish we are to have lost sight of the religious importance of dreams! But what good are they?

First, dreams give us perspective. Oftentimes a problem will seem overwhelming and unsolvable. When we "sleep on" the problem, our dreams frequently give us our unconscious answer. When we wake up from such dreams, we simply know the right decision to make.

Second, our dreams force us to deal with repressed areas of our life. Everything that has ever happened to us is stuffed way down inside somewhere. In our waking hours the repressed memories never make it to the surface. But in our dreams we are forced to deal with these sensitive areas so that our mental health can be maintained.

Third, dreams help us discover how unfairly and subjectively we treat others. We learn this by paying attention to the persons who appear in our dreams. In almost every instance we are really not dreaming about other persons at all; we are often actually dreaming about ourselves. The other persons in our dreams only represent aspects of our own personality. By observing what labels and stereotypes we unconsciously lay on other persons, we can learn to treat them more fairly when we are awake.

Fourth, dreams are sometimes vehicles for ESP. Have you ever had a premonition in a dream? Apparently millions of Americans have had them. In the spiritual realm, ordinary chronological time does not exist. A dream may well warn us of an impending disaster or future occurrence. Let it be noted, by the way, that no one professes to understand fully how all this works.

Finally, in certain "breakthrough" dreams we get not just

perspective on our problems but major spiritual insights. The key is in knowing how to interpret the dreams.

Have you ever had a dream about falling through space? Drowning? Being chased and unable to move your legs? Being pursued by a sinister figure? Being locked in a room? Dancing? Making love? Being lost in the woods? Caught in quicksand?

One should beware of simplistic interpretations of dreams; a qualified therapist is always needed to investigate the precise significance that the individual should attach to the image in the dream. But the chances are that if you have ever had any variation of the dreams listed above, you have been told something about yourself that is very important spiritually.

To the best of my knowledge, the Catholic Church has almost totally abdicated its interest in dream interpretation to professional psychiatrists. This is bad news for two reasons: Our religious myths and symbols can offer a veritable gold mine in helping persons come to terms with their dreams; and many, if not most, psychiatrists have no time at all for religion.

Dream interpretation is another area in which church-related persons simply have to take more interest. To ignore that part of our lives is to cut off a potentially great source of spiritual growth.

What's in a Dream?

Everyone dreams every night from four to seven times. Whether or not we remember our dreams is beside the point; these nightly occurrences do in fact play a significant role in our lives.

What do dreams do for us? They have a very definite healing effect because in our dreams we work out many of the conflicts we are either unwilling or unable to deal with on a conscious level.

But how do dreams fit in with the Christian perspective? Actually they are very compatible, even though this whole area has been largely avoided in the religious education of most of us.

Just page through the Old and New Testaments and notice how often dreams are the means by which persons realized what they should be doing with their lives. Sometimes they were convinced that God himself had spoken to them in dreams.

But Catholics cannot just stop with the Scriptures. What does our tradition say about it? Interestingly enough, every major father in the early church, from Justin Martyr to Cyprian, believed that individuals could receive genuine spiritual revelation through dreams. The same opinion was held by Athanasius, Ambrose, Augustine, and many other doctors of the church. Let's get down to the business of sharing this part of our Catholic spiritual heritage.

What do we dream about? Let us take a quick and admittedly simplified look. We dream on roughly eight different levels.

Level one: We dream about things in our recent memory. It may be about some event that just took place.

Level two: We sometimes dream about things that happened to us in the past, incidents that we have completely suppressed from our conscious thought. These are events that are too painful to remember when we are awake.

Level three: Sometimes we have a dream that seems to have nothing to do with anything that has ever happened to us before. Such dreams can give us pointed insights in making major life-decisions.

Level four: We occasionally have dreams that are filled with universal symbols. We seem to be born with these common symbols. Some such symbols that may crop up in our dreams are the ocean, a stranger, a wise old man, or a dark forest.

Level five: Persons sometimes wake up with a clear conviction that someone or something has communicated to them some needed advice and direction. This is one reason why some persons want to sleep on a problem before making a final decision.

Level six: Persons in dreams sometimes have the experience of a powerful encounter with either goodness or evil—an encounter either very encouraging or very frightening.

Level seven: Some dreams provide a sudden intuition. Great music, poetry, and scientific discoveries have been scribbled down by individuals who awake in the middle of the night with the conviction that they had been inspired by a dream.

Level eight: Some fortunate individuals have a dream in which the true nature of reality is revealed to them. Such a dream can permanently affect a person's life for the good.

Run for Your Life

Isn't it a blessing when someone comes up with an activity that can improve our physical, mental, and spiritual well-being? Millions of Americans have found such an activity: running (or jogging).

Soft, paunchy, and pale Americans walking around today are the "beneficiaries" of improved technology. Machines do practically everything for us. Consequently, most of us are only one emotional trauma away from dropping dead at any time.

Running has been amply demonstrated to improve one's physical health. This is no longer even debated. A regular program of running has been shown to improve one's cardiorespiratory endurance, muscular endurance, strength, balance, weight control, muscle definition, digestion, and sleep.

Of course, the price tag for all these benefits is the discipline of working out and following an organized program for oneself. This does not go over so well with those Americans who, according to Dr. John H. Knowles, president of the Rockefeller Foundation, regard "sloth, gluttony, alcoholic intemperance, reckless driving, sexual frenzy, and smoking as constitutional rights."

Some such folks probably have an unconscious "death wish" and consider taking care of their bodies a waste of time. But for those who enjoy feeling better, running should be given serious consideration.

The benefits are not just physical, however. Running seems to improve one's mental outlook as well. Some psychiatrists are suggesting running as an antidote to anxiety and depression. Some doctors are recommending it as a "positive addiction" for alcoholics. The average person frequently experiences profound mental changes as a result of running.

As one friend of mine told me, "I've only been jogging for a couple of weeks, but I already feel that I'm seeing things with better perspective. Things seem less cluttered. I feel as if my mind has more space in it."

Runners also seem to acquire more energy. The afternoon is the time when I begin to "fade." It would seem a natural remedy for me to lie down and take a nap. But when instead I force myself to head to the park for a half-hour run, it is almost as if I am "reborn." I can face my evening appointments with a clear and rested mind and with a surplus of energy. I do not know how all this works, but I do know that it works.

But, perhaps most interestingly of all, there are also spiritual benefits to running. Michael Murphy, the founder of Esalen, thinks many runners are "closet mystics." I agree with him. When two runners begin comparing notes, there is often some mention made of a "transcendental high" or mystical breakthrough experienced while running.

All religions speak of the necessity of losing oneself. Something like this often happens to runners. Unexpectedly they experience themselves as part of a process greater than themselves. While running, they lose that sense of self-consciousness that plagues us all, and they experience themselves flowing rhythmically with nature.

Another spiritual benefit of running is that it can facilitate meditation. I personally find it almost impossible to pray while in the parish rectory. It seems that the phone or doorbell is ringing eighteen hours a day. Even if it does not ring when I am trying to pray, I am still distracted because I am aware that it might ring. I am sure that roughly the same situation prevails in many other households.

There are no phones or doorbells in the woods. One can

really let one's mind and spirit loose and sometimes be flooded with a sense of God's presence. One day while jogging my mind started making spiritual connections. When I returned home, I outlined five pages of how God's plan fits together. This might have happened while I was praying in church or somewhere else. But it happened while I was jogging.

The only way to find out if running can do all these things for you is to give it an honest try. You may find, as I did, that running will help you physically, mentally, and spiritually.

Children of Light

The influence of light on the human being can hardly be overestimated. Just as plants and trees lean toward the sun, so human beings have an innate need for natural light.

According to Dr. Margaret Cleaves, sunlight stimulates nerve terminals in the skin and actually increases our energy. That is why we usually feel better and more energized in the summer than we do in the winter. In addition, sunlight releases a special hormone that improves the functioning of our muscles and sense organs. All things being equal, people who are exposed to the sunlight will be healthier than individuals who live and work in dark surroundings or in artificial lighting.

It is important that the light we receive be as natural as possible. Most of us spend much of our time in artificially illuminated environments. As John Ott, director of the Environmental Health and Light Research Institute, puts it, our time is spent "behind window glass and windshield, watching TV, looking through colored sunglasses, working in window-less buildings . . . ." He points out that most glass filters out the natural light and that many human ills are attributable to living in such an artificial environment.

If a person is actually absorbing light, and if this light is having a positive effect on the person, then is it possible to measure the amount of light a person has assimilated? Yes, it is. All forms of nature emit wavelengths called auras.

The first person to measure scientifically the light fields around humans was Dr. Walter Kilner of England. Back in the early 1900s, he found that auras could be measured through glass screens colored with certain types of dyes. He found that human beings have scientifically measurable auras extending as much as eight inches around the body. Furthermore, the auras were comprised of different colors that could be influenced by fatigue or disease.

The measuring of this force field was simplified by Valentina Kirlian and her husband Samyon Kirlian. These Russian researchers developed a form of photography that captures the sparks, flashes, and small explosions that are constantly being emitted by our bodies. Blue, green, gold, and violet colors emanate from us all.

Although few of us have the psychic gift to see auras, many more are able to sense, if not see, the force fields of other persons. Even before another person says anything to us it is sometimes rather easy to sense whether he or she is healthy or sick, happy or sad, spiritual or materialistic, loving or egocentric.

This business about auras should not be entirely strange to us Christians. After all, our saints have almost always been portrayed with haloes over their heads. Was this just the artist's imagination? Have not spiritually enlightened persons always been surrounded by beautiful auras?

When Jesus called us children of light, he may have been saying something about us that is literally true, in a different sense. We flourish in the light and wither in the darkness. Deprive our bodies of the sunlight and we court disease. Deprive our souls of the inner light found in prayer and we become trapped in depression and self-hatred. As children of the light, our heritage and birthright is the fullness of physical and spiritual health.

Positive Thinking

One of the most important steps in gaining mental and spiritual health is the systematic elimination of negative thinking. It is not enough just to cleanse our house of unruly devils, however. We must replace the old ways of thinking with positive thoughts.

Jesus spoke about the value of belief. It is necessary to believe *in advance* that there is a God and that life is worthwhile and that we are all fundamentally good. You begin with the conclusions and, in time, you eventually discover that it all makes sense.

We make a leap of faith that we have a lot to do with determining our fate. We then accept in faith the premise that life and human beings are basically good, and we live and think accordingly. The results can be amazing. Sounds too good to be true, does it? But the fact of the matter is that it works. It is something like a psychosomatic illness in reverse. Our positive thinking eventually leads us toward mental and spiritual health.

We may think this is all a lot of nonsense because we have become so locked into the vicious cycle of negative thinking. We prefer the darkness to the light because we have forgotten what the light even looks like.

Maybe we came from families where we were always "put down" by our parents or ridiculed by our brothers and sisters. We were told that we were "good for nothing" for so long in so many subtle and overt ways that we eventually began to believe it. We became trapped in a cycle of negativity.

If we are fortunate enough to realize there is an alternative to this miserable way to exist, we are on the road to recovery. We then stubbornly insist on replacing (not repressing) the negative, destructive thoughts with positive, healthful ones.

At first the process is slow. Especially when we are alone, the old tapes begin to play again. Self-pity, guilt, recrimination, self-hate—all the old devils—try to regain a foothold in our interior mansion. But we sweep them away again by the power of the risen Christ.

According to Carl Jung, the Catholic Church has an amazingly sophisticated set of symbols that, used properly, can contribute to mental health. Unlike some other religious groups, we do not adopt a Pollyanna approach to the human condition. We fully accept our originally sinful condition. But then we must go beyond the fall to Calvary.

If we can enter into the life of Jesus and die with him, we will also rise with him. As Christians, we are given a full charge of His risen Spirit. If we can enter fully into the church's liturgical year, we cannot help but become an Easter people, a people with a positive, healthy outlook.

Why, then, are so many seemingly religious persons so glum and downcast? There are probably all sorts of hereditary, environmental, and mental factors for this behavior. But one thing is for sure. Everything we need for a positive outlook on life is found within the traditions of our faith.

Reclaiming Our Lives

Medicine treats the body apart from the mind and spirit. Psychology treats the mind apart from the body and spirit. And the churches treat the spirit apart from the body and the mind. Where is wholeness?

Technology proliferates with no moral considerations. Society tries to deal with issues without considering the religious dimension. And the religions blissfully ignore everything except their own self-interests. Where is wholeness?

At first glance, it looks like our society is still completely compartmentalized. But when we look deeper, we see that a quiet revolution is brewing. Author Marilyn Ferguson refers to this revolution as the "Aquarian Conspiracy." It is a revolution without leaders and without dogmas. Its underlying principle is a belief in a wholistic vision of our universe. This revolution has conspirators in the government, private industry, medicine, education, the military, and the churches.

There is nothing insidious about this revolution. No foreign government will be taking over anyone else. What we are talking about is a revolution whereby people are regaining control over their own lives. We are realizing that we are the earth and the earth is us and we all have the responsibility to be co-evolvers with God.

In the past, we often deferred to the great institutions of society to run our lives for us. Government made all the decisions affecting the direction of our country for us. The schools taught our children; our military took care of defending us; doctors looked after our bodies; and the churches took care of our souls. After years of living with this sort of compartmentalization, we are reaping the whirlwind of living fragmented lives. Government bureaucracies are out of control; our schools are sometimes graduating illiterates; modern medicine treats us like machines instead of persons; our military has us in a position of being thirty minutes from doomsday; and our churches have lost touch with their spiritual wisdom.

People are now in the process of reclaiming control over their lives. This is what wholeness is about. Never again will we abdicate our personal responsibility and defer to institutions that "know better" than we do.

Certainly it is adolescent romanticism to believe that we can do without our great institutions. They can serve us greatly as extensions of ourselves, but institutions are there to serve us and not the other way around.

There is really nothing new in all this. The very word "holiness" comes from the Greek word that means "wholeness." In its origins and in its finest moments, the church always realized that to be holy meant to be whole. Somewhere along the line we just forgot.

Today we are in the process of reclaiming this wholistic view of life. We want some say and some responsibility in all the major decisions affecting our lives. Whether we chalk it up to Aquarius or the Holy Spirit, certainly we live in amazing times. We live in a great period of transition, a time when we are waking up to our awesome responsibility to ourselves, to future generations, and to the planet itself. I can think of no greater time to be alive.